Your Best Health by Friday

*How to Overcome Anxiety, Depression, Stress, Trauma,
PTSD and Chronic Illness*

By

Elizabeth Gould
M.S.

Printed in the United States of America.

First Printing: October, 2017
Rincon Star Press

This book is not intended to be a substitute for the medical advice of a licensed physician. The reader
should consult with their doctor in any matters related to his/her health.

ISBN 978-1-387-33463-6

Praise for Your Best Health by Friday

The US Review of Books
reviewed by Megan Bain

"If you are anxious, depressed or chronically ill, please don't be discouraged about where you are."

This practical guide contains research on reducing chronic illness. These recommendations are to aid readers' medical plans. This simple plan is divided into five days of learning. Monday describes ways to reduce stress. Tuesday outlines understanding pain. Wednesday teaches how to stop reliving negative emotions that cloud your mind. Thursday stresses ways to develop breathing practices to control emotions, exercise, and how to use vision and thoughts to heal. Finally, Friday discusses how the digestive system and diet work together to aid your body in retaining nutrients needed for overall health.

Gould has lived with chronic illness her whole life due to a multitude of unfortunate circumstances. These illnesses had her on multiple medications, but the side effects were just as bad as the illness itself. Gould chose to start researching alternatives to modern medicine to heal her body, instead of just masking the troubles with medication. She shares her experiences in the hope of helping others in her situation. While Gould addresses the main issues of most individuals living with a chronic illness, she takes what doctors describe and breaks it down in ways the readers can understand. At the end of each day's lesson, she even demonstrates ways the reader can start using this information by organizing ideas into easy, moderate, and harder steps so no reader is overwhelmed when starting this regimen. She emphasizes that no one should start all the steps at once, but take a few actions toward a healthier way to heal one's body and when comfortable, add more. Gould has designed a simple, researched way to help readers heal and experience a better life.

Through her research, Gould has designed a simple way to help her readers heal and experience a better life. By sharing her personal experiences from childhood to adulthood, Gould builds a rapport with her readers developing a trust in her knowledge of the subject. Throughout the book, she references other authors' works which she uses as a guide to her own course of action lending sincerity to her study and ideas. Within each lesson, she directs her readers to other sites, books, and studies in order for the reader to learn more

3

about the techniques and practices that most interest them and will fit best within their lifestyle never promoting that her way is the best or only way, thus showing the reader genuineness from Gould proving she is truly sharing her experiences simply to help her readers gain a healthier, less painful, and more fulfilling lifestyle.

RECOMMENDED by the US Review

The following is an email I received from the reviewer, which I include in this book with her permission:

Subject: Your Best Health by Friday
Date: December 20, 2017 at 10:45:34 AM
To: <elizabeth@rightbrainuniversity.com>
From: Megan Bain

I am not sure if this email will find Elizabeth Gould, *Your Best Health by Friday* author, but I hope it does. This is the reviewer from US Book Review. I have never felt the need to contact an author before, but I must tell you this book spoke directly to me. I had been a teacher since 1999. Last December, I had to quit and was put on disability due to my fibromyalgia. I am 40, feel sad all the time due to my illness, and miss a lot of my children's events due to illness. I cannot wait to try the steps in your book. I feel like that review was sent to me by a higher power. I was meant to read your inspiring words. Thank you for letting me review your book. Not only did I get to review it, but I also get to grow from it which is something that has never happened before in my reviews. Thank you for sharing your personal experiences and research so those of us with this condition can relieve some pain, stress, and depression. I will be using all of your suggestions and just want to thank you for sharing this with the world so we can use your years of research and start healing now.

Thanks,
Megan

Dedication:

to Michael, for believing
to Alex & Dylan, for being

Acknowledgements

To my friends for putting up with my one track mind over the years:-) Jan Ottmann, Rachelle Gebler, Joanne Johnson, Ina Hamilton, Robyn Holden Geach, Jan Atkinson, Barbe Crowley, Betsy Sawyer, Bobbi Buttonow, Carol White Llewellyn, Staci and Chris Skelly, Cindy Brokaw, Ellen Paltiel, Lisa Fleischauer, Jen Ross, Jaime Echt, Vera Zamdmer, Tobi Harlukowicz, Karen Altabef, Louise Lahiff O'Sullivan, Mitch Sylves-Berry, Nancy Checchi, Phyllis Arduino, Mary Lazin, Roberta Straus, Sanderia Smith, Senia Sakaria, Stephanie Ortiz, Nancy D'Aurizio, Amy Demner, and Susan Allor.

In appreciation to my family: Michael, Alex and Dylan, Pop, Becky, Ricki, Dwain, Kate, Ian, Adam, Simon and Nicola, Cat, Mike, Kira and Gavin.

To my mom, Jan Wharton, for starting me on the path and to Oprah Winfrey for being a guiding light with *What I Know For Sure*.

With thanks to Dr. James Roach, Dr. John Douillard, Dr. Valerie Girard, Dr. Sara Whitney, Dr. Lizzie Clapham, Matthew Thie, M.Ed., Hazel Gale, Dr. Anne Jensen, and Paula Oleska.

Deep thanks to another dear friend and author, Chad Cryder, for your wit, wisdom and encouragement.

My mentors Julie Newendorp and Annegret Wolf Rice, who helped me build a life worth living.

To two standout therapists who've helped me integrate mind and body, Alan Levin and Cheryle Van Scoy.

To my writing partner, Marcia Meier, founder of Weeping Willow Press, for your help, talent and kindness.

To my Toastmasters group, Mission Toastmasters of Santa Barbara, for all your encouragement.

and huge thanks to Steve Harrison and Geoffrey Berwin of Quantum Leap as well as to Ann McIndoo, my author's coach.

Table of Contents

Friday: Improve Digestion and Nutrient Absorption

Introduction

This book is written for people who think their best years are behind them, like I once did. If you've struggled your whole life to overcome your past, if you're chronically stressed, if you've let anxiety and depression make your world small, if you've suffered from poor health or chronic illness, it's not too late to rebuild your health. I've done it, and maybe if you try some of what I've tried you could be healthier and happier too.

I set out to learn how to be braver for my children's sakes, but what I discovered was that learning freedom from fear of my emotions freed my spiritual side. This in turn led to freedom from my thoughts, which then led to freedom from my physical illness. I've tried to organize my process into lessons in the hope that others who might want a shortcut may follow. As always, it's entirely up to you what your life journey is about.

It seems to me that when we don't listen to what our body needs and what our life's purpose is, it leads to our getting sick. We can develop lasting beliefs about ourselves from our childhoods which live on as unconscious programming and run counter to our optimal health. I believe the body heals itself when we examine and release these old holdings and start living with integrity towards our needs and life's purpose. Many of us live a life so tied to the mind that we have very little opportunity for emotional, physical or spiritual development. It's possible to get a taste of what others experience in these other areas—-and by so doing increase our sense of happiness and fulfillment—-while remaining true to our core sense of self and beliefs. I'll show you how I've made my life happier and healthier thanks to examining the mind.

I tried living a small, sheltered life to avoid my anxieties, but they found me anyway. Chronic illness—fibromyalgia—found me too.

I'm just an everyday person who wouldn't give up trying to heal myself. I've also learned the hard way how to rebound and rebuild, as well as the commonalities to all sorts of illnesses, so you don't have to waste another day living with what appears to be your lot in life. Start turning your life around with these fixes. I'm going to simply explain some things so that you may understand what gets us into this mess. Then I'll divide the information into five lessons—which I've listed under the five days of the week—and tools to learn them. Once you understand the lessons, you can check in anytime you want to make sure you've incorporated them into your daily life, and if you haven't, reset your intentions.

I'll offer suggestions for things you can do to help yourself. If you're mostly healthy, keep things simple and try the easiest version. If you're sick, you might want to go deeper. Dip a toe in—and please don't try to make too many changes at once. One thing at a time. These are all things I learned over the course of the past 10 years. If I'd done them all at once, I'd have fried my circuit board.

The lessons:

Monday	*Reduce Stress, Increase Flow*
Tuesday	*Understand Pain*
Wednesday	*Stop Reliving Emotions*
Thursday	*Develop Parasympathetic Breathing, Exercise, Vision and Thoughts*
Friday	*Improve Digestion and Nutrient Absorption*

If you are anxious, depressed or chronically ill, please don't be discouraged about where you are. You can, if you choose, learn to be encouraged about where you are going. The power of intention is very strong. You may open a book like this and think that you have no hope of changing. Your thought creates an intention that you will not change, though, so try to be open to change; at a minimum, try to reserve your opinion. Thinking is so often judging and judging is so often negative. It holds us captive. To change this, whenever I catch myself judging, I imagine a green heart outline around the thing or person that I've harmed through my thoughts so I can see them in a kinder way.

If you find yourself impatient, anxious or blue, remember that this is a sign that your left brain is kicking in. It's a sign that you've got an expectation——because it is only with expectation and judgment that we or others in our life fall short. It's never okay to accept an abusive situation, but if I know I am safe and loved, I find it helpful to learn to accept what is——and find the love for what is through my struggles and doubts. I walk in nature or use a diluted essential oil like pine or eucalyptus to bring me back to expansion, hope and mental calm. I often meditate at these times. Prayer works well, if you are open to it. Feel yourself letting stress melt away. Then loop back to the beginning, to the intention of where you're going. However much you've strayed from the path, accept what is. Think kind and loving thoughts about yourself for trying. You'll grow your ability to stay on the path by checking in with intention frequently. Always remember though, that this is a journey. We aren't expected to be perfect, just that we try to make progress. Underneath it all, we'll find love at the core of our being.

I was, am, and expect to be challenged every day of my life for as long as I am growing. I choose to grow despite the fear of pushing through. This is because I've learned that if I give up, disease, pain, despair and hopelessness await. I've been there and I don't want to go back. Now my destination is health, well-being, happiness, expansion and joy.

I hope you find useful information in this book, but remember that you are the expert in your own life. Perhaps someone has pressured you to read this book and none of this feels like the right fit for you. That's okay. You always have the right to choose to do none of what I suggest. That's a decision you get to make. I've created action steps in case anyone wants to try what I've done, but I always defer to the reader as being their own best guide. There are many pathways to health. Perhaps seeing what has worked for me can help

you have your best health and happiest life yet; perhaps not. Either
way, I am always cheering you on.

Love,
Elizabeth

Chapter 1
How Chronic Stress Kills

Outer Chronic Stress

We likely think of stress as being a bad thing and that chronic stress is even worse. Stress is any situation that motivates us to act or change, and as such, it can be neutral, good or bad. Hunger is an example of a stress and feeding ourselves the right amount of healthy food is a good outcome.

Outer chronic stress is when we have the motivation to act or change our environment but for some reason we feel unable to do so; whether it is because of external conditions in our lives, like being repressed in some way during our childhood years, or needing to keep our job in order to pay our mortgage.

Inner Chronic Stress

We put a lot of pressure on ourselves with negative self-talk and how we think about ourselves. This is inner chronic stress.

Inner chronic stress can be the most insidious because we often believe that without constantly pushing ourselves we will be lazy or useless and amount to nothing. So many of us have a streak of perfectionism that constantly beats up our inner child, our unconscious self.

We harangue and berate ourselves at times to win the love and approval of our parents, teachers and friends, and it can become a habit because it seems to have worked in the past. Because it is self-generated, it is easily turned around, however we must learn to listen to how we speak to ourselves:

"I'm such an idiot!"

"Dad was right; I'm a failure"

"I'll never lose this weight!"

Children Want to Please

I believe that we need to understand that most children are born eager to please. If children are given love and positive encouragement along with tools to help with self-discovery and personal growth, they will develop a balance between being true to themselves and their calling, as well as finding joy in making others happy.

Children are often taught more by the unconscious teachings of the adults in their lives through nonverbal communications rather than by the verbal. It's said that most of communication happens nonverbally. As parents, we are often unaware of what we "say" nonverbally. The emotional stress that we feel when our children are up all night with a fever, and then bounce back, while we suffer from lack of sleep, can result in overreaction to our children's behavior.

Even if we do not overreact visibly, the stress we feel is in our brain state. This helps explain why our kids often start to act out when we are having a bad day. In addition to biochemical cues, I believe they are reacting to the painful feelings from their mirror neurons caused by our own emotional state, and they do not know what to do about it.

Similarly, I think we react to our children's distress, anger and fear because it is generated unconsciously within our mirror neurons when we see it in them. How nice it would be to have the skills to reset our emotional state so we do not have to keep reacting to each other in a negative way when we are having a bad day.

Our Unconscious Mind Runs the Show Under our Noses

Our unconscious beliefs are not easy to access, but they drive most of our behavior. Most of those patterns and beliefs were formed before we were six-years-old, according to molecular biologists such as Dr. Bruce Lipton of Stanford. I don't know about you, but I am uncomfortable at the thought that most of my behavior is being run by that childhood self of mine.

Adverse Childhood Experience (ACE) Test

I first heard about the ACE test in 2015 from an NPR piece. For those who haven't heard of it, doctors have realized that traumatic events from our childhood increase risk factors for poor health in later life. The likelihood of our having problems with issues as diverse as smoking, drug and alcohol abuse, missing work, obesity, diabetes, heart disease, cancer, depression, suicide attempts, and COPD (chronic obstructive pulmonary disorder) increases based on how traumatic our childhoods were. Things like abuse, neglect and household dysfunction impact us long after our childhoods are over. As Donna Jackson Nakazawa reports in *Childhood Disrupted*, "chronic stress leads to dysregulation of our stress hormones, which leads to unregulated inflammation. And inflammation translates into symptoms and disease." Many other factors go into whether we will get sick, but the right hemisphere of the brain doesn't have a sense of time. Until the emotions from these traumatic events are processed and released, they are stored in our body and we will continue to suffer. I've included the ACE test in the back of this book in the Appendix. In addition to answering these questions for yourself, I suggest you think about how your parents would answer these questions, as well as your grandparents. I think it has a bearing that I'll go into later in the book. It's clear that what we don't face from our childhoods is contributing to us getting sick, which gave me a great deal of motivation to look back at those early years.

Why I Needed Healing

I was born into a military family during the Vietnam War, while my dad was on active duty in Vietnam. His combat stress translated into PTSD for me. It doesn't take much to put babies into a freeze state that is easily re-triggered. My unconscious patterns brought nothing but increasing amounts of fear, restriction, isolation, and ultimately pain from Fibromyalgia.

Fibromyalgia feels like an overloaded circuit board that is about to ignite. To give an example, if my body were a house, it'd be a house with all the lights on, all the appliances running, everything churning, grinding and wearing out. I needed to find help. I had been frozen in a state of chronic stress for over 40 years and I was about to discover the consequences. I needed answers before it was too late.

Medication gave me too many side effects to deal with. I needed to find the root of my problems so I could heal.

Chapter 2
How the Brain Works

The Three Layers of the Brain

The newest part of the human brain is the outermost layer and is called the cortex. The part behind our forehead is called the prefrontal cortex. The second oldest part generates our emotions and it is the middle layer; it is called the limbic system or the emotional brain.

The oldest part is at the base of the skull, closest to the top of the spine and continues into the spinal cord. It is called the primitive or reptilian brain and controls the autonomic nervous system (ANS).

Left/Right Handshake

There are two sides to the brain, called hemispheres. Their jobs are not so delineated as we've been told, but I'll stick with that model to keep it simple. The left side is mostly in charge of the academic: things like writing, math and language and words. The right-side deals with the creative, but is also in charge of processing unconscious data, whether it is social, emotional, or sensory information.

Since most of our brain capacity is unconscious, the right side of the brain is important. The right brain handles our sensory processing: vision, smell, taste, touch, hearing, balance (this is called the vestibular system, which is based in the inner ear), as well as internal sensations such as the feedback from our body as it sits in a chair. These internal sensations of gravity are called the proprioceptive system. The proprioceptive system is responsible for taking the input from our senses and acting on them to keep us safe.

The right brain is also in charge of processing all nonverbal communication, which accounts for the majority of the communicating we do. This means it oversees our social success. For those who have high functioning autistic spectrum issues, key areas of the right brain are underdeveloped and can't process the social input fast enough, so the information is ignored. The right brain also processes information connected to heart rate, breathing, blood pressure, digestion, body temperature and metabolism. The left brain does a vitally important job: the logical thinking, verbal, analytical, math and writing skills that are all critical. It makes sure we eat and are productive so we as individuals survive. It has a voice—it is our conscious self, and it makes its needs known, often very insistently.

The right brain is always plugging along as the silent partner whose needs are ignored, or at best, the last ones met. Lots of us are Type-A workaholics who ignore impulses to play or are so busy being responsible adults that we shame ourselves into disconnecting from our creative passions.

For our Best Health, both Mental and Physical

For perfect health, we need both sides of our brain to be fully developed because they need to work together. For example, many of the functions of the immune system and digestive system need to be cross-coordinated. The digestive tract is muscle-based and needs to be able to hand off from the muscles of the right half of the body to those on the left half of the body as food does its dance through the intestinal tract.

If we have one hemisphere that is underdeveloped, it is not possible to have an optimal digestive system. This is because the nutrients necessary for building and repairing our body are only provided by a healthy, fully developed left and right brain so that we have optimal digestion.

Every step of the process of food being absorbed, and of the body being able to repair the digestive tract requires a balanced brain.

It's also not possible to have an optimal immune system if one hemisphere is underdeveloped because both hemispheres control its proper functioning.

I think of the brain as being in a lifelong three-legged race. If we think back to those in a three-legged race, it wasn't the children paired with the adults (an underdeveloped hemisphere paired with a fully developed one) who won. The winners were a pair of adults with similar leg length and had experience at matching rhythm in day-to-day life.

When we are stressed, we use our dominant hemisphere, which is the most developed. This gives us the fastest reaction time possible to get away from a predator. In modern times, the stress might be taking a test or giving a presentation at work. For example, if our dominant hemisphere is the right brain (which does not house words or math), we can imagine just how much of a handicap that would be. People with a dominant right hemisphere often have a problem with text anxiety.

There are always connections to the opposite hemisphere so it is not like we often go completely blank, but for some people it can get close.

The Power of Repetitive Movement

Learning begins with something called our primary, also known as primitive, reflexes. Primary reflexes are a way that babies automatically start learning about the world; these reflexes start in utero and build on each other. Each type of primary reflex is supposed to start at a specific age and last for a certain number of months. These time-tested patterns of movement allow synapses to make vital connections. They also allow development of the fatty sheath coating called myelin that gets laid down around a motor neuron every time it is used, which helps signal travel through it faster.

Signals can travel up to five times faster through myelinated neurons than unmyelinated ones. The faster the signals travel, the faster we can process information and our reactions. The more myelin coating, the stronger our grip will be.

IQ is a Measure of Processing Speed

Since IQ is a measure of processing speed among other factors, the thicker (and therefore stronger) the myelin sheath, the better we can perform on IQ tests. Myelin destruction is common in many central nervous system disorders like Parkinson's disease and Multiple Sclerosis. Repetitive movement is the key to the development of healthy amounts of myelin. The brain is efficient at pruning unused connections. If we have not used a connection in seven years, it is gone. If we haven't frequently balanced with our eyes closed, ridden a bike or taken dance classes in a long enough time, we will notice a decline in our ability to balance. I believe the mental decline that some people experience as they age is largely because they move less, challenge their balance less and therefore the thinking process is happening on a slower circuit as there is less and less myelin coating.

Brain Growth Through Challenging Balance

Many of us think we maintain good balance by running, but running presents a limited challenge to our brain. Running challenges our forward balance, but provides limited challenge to our balance going backwards, up, down and side to side. Different parts of our brain handle each of these types of movement. The more we repeat a movement the more synaptic connections are made and the more dendrites (short branched extensions of nerve cells) are made. It's all brain growth, and that's a huge positive for us.

Myelin is added to a part of the neuron called the axon so that the whole system is in peak working order. If you have not been good about cross training in yoga or dance and you are in your thirties or older, hold onto a counter and close your eyes. Cautiously let go and see how good your balance is, then stand on your tiptoes and sink into a crouch and stand up. Chances are it is more of an effort than it used to be. Now try challenging yourself by asking a friend to spot you, so you do not fall. Can you close your eyes, bend over and touch your toes? Can you close your eyes, stand on your tiptoes and turn around with good balance or are you shaky?

Couch potatoes can see trouble with this at a much younger age. It's part of the slippery slope that leads so many people to using walkers or wheelchairs at far too young an age. Fear of losing their balance leads to people further restricting their activity which only accelerates the decline. Restricting activity means not producing as much myelin. This will make movement and balance become ever more challenging.

It is never too late. My eighty-four-year-old father took up yoga three years ago and he loves it. He has gone from being unable to get up on his own if he fell (he had double knee replacement surgery ten years ago and never regained full mobility afterwards), to now easily being able to get up. He's much more limber, active and happy.

Our Left-Brain Culture

It is my belief that as a society we overly value the left brain. Our education system targets the left brain. Any problems that we experience in learning are addressed by strengthening our left-brain abilities.

Our children are expected to sit at a desk and learn to read at younger and younger ages with each passing generation. They are often punished for not conforming by having their freedom to play taken away, by being held in at recess. There is also less and less time for free play allowed for children, both at home and at school. Children receive less self-directed playtime; learning has a schedule and young minds are constantly turned to academic goals.

Developing Children's Right Brains

Scheduled play dates that often center around video games do not allow for developing the right brain. The primitive brain cannot tell the difference between real and imagined images so all the gaming produces adrenaline, the same feeling as if the player were firing a gun in real life.

One of the big prerequisites for developing the right brain is the willingness to let children get bored so they can go inward and discover what causes them to begin practicing creative play rather than just being consumers of entertainment. Our left-brain culture has made academic learning the only priority. School tests are designed to test the left brain, so it appears that accentuating left-brain learning produces more concrete academic success, however the right brain is invaluable for seeing the big picture and being able to focus attention, among other things. (While it has long been associated with creativity, and the left hemisphere with logic, the best examples of creativity and logic come from the whole brain functioning together.)

Bringing Back Music, Art and Daily P.E.

In many schools, physical education is only two or three days a week for one semester of the year. Students stand in lines, bored, as they wait for instruction on how to play a game, rather than staying active in a game and getting pulled out for instructional game training. One suggestion is to let kids use a jump rope while they wait. In elementary school, punishment for the bad behavior of one child is often taking away recess time for an entire class.

There are fewer art and music teachers and often entire music programs have been eliminated. The right brain learns through movement, art, music and creativity. It is how we find flow (the state in which we are fully immersed in a feeling of energized focus, full involvement and enjoyment in an activity) and get back in balance when we suffer from too much thinking, which tires us out and floods us with stress hormones.

Small wonder we are stressed, small wonder high school and college students report a lack of joy in their lives. It seems logical to believe this lack of joy and hope could cause a rise in suicide rates.

Surrendering Ego can be Difficult in Our Search for Help

Because of school and societal emphasis, we likely have a more developed left brain than right brain. The downside of our logical, rational left brain is that it is constantly judging. If we are always in that state, there is no peace. Our right brain specializes in non-judgmental processing. When we are in that state, we are peaceful. Our stress can reset to calm. Many of us reach the limits of how much our left brain can help us at some point in our lives. We spiral into anxiety or depression and do not know how to reorder our thoughts so that we don't keep spiraling downward. Using the right brain to reset to calm is not something we're taught in school, and it's often not something we're taught at home either.

Too much thinking, in and of itself, can be a big part of the problem. Overthinking leads to over-feeling and vice versa, both of which often fly beneath our conscious radar. This causes a release of chemicals in our body. Neurons in our brain release neuropeptides to communicate with other neurons. When we are very upset, too much thinking can generate too many neuropeptides, giving us a kind of woozy emotional hangover that can feel like having too much to drink. We often get caught in a negative thought loop where a negative thought can scare our unconscious, which then causes fear and anxiety, which in turn scares us consciously until we have another negative thought. It's a downward spiral. Unless we acknowledge the thoughts and feelings, we remain caught in the loop and the neuropeptides persist in our body. The neuropeptides are created by our emotional (limbic) brain, and are meant to increase our chance of survival, so they never release until we process and learn from them. Unfortunately, when they're stored they cause inflammation in our body, which leads to illness.

Beyond the Ego-Self

That dominant left brain keeps us locked into our ego, our lonely self, and prevents us from engaging the right brain, which processes all the nonverbal social cues. I think most of us are wired to be at peace when we are in community, despite whatever traumas might keep us from consciously feeling comfortable in community. When our right brain is more active we can see the big picture and how wonderful it is to be alive, even in the worst of times.

Our left brain is for the survival of the self. Our right brain is for connection to others. How ironic that too much self-thinking can spiral into thoughts of ending the self because we cannot bear the pain of the self when the self feels alone and abandoned.

Celebrate Every Baby Step towards Developing the Right Brain

Many of us have had some sense of having a gut feeling or intuition at some point in our lives. This is a part of the right brain talking to us. The more we acknowledge and act on our gut feelings, the more that window opens to us.

We are Body/Mind—the Heart and the Gut Also Must be Heard

We have neurons in three areas of our body: the mind, gut and heart. All three need to be in harmony. I've learned the hard way that health flies out the door when they are not. That part of our brain that we know of as ourselves is only a small fraction of our whole self; our ego self is not in charge.

Once Body and Mind are in Sync, Health can be Rebuilt

I have been humbled enough by life's circumstances to realize that my conscious self is not in charge of my life. My unconscious is the bigger part and my ego self can only try to act as a guide to that unconscious. I realize it is a lifelong process to parent my unconscious self. I must think of my greater good, of the positive way of communicating to myself. It's been my habit of negative communication with my unconscious that brought problems and disease into my life.

I noticed that once I could catch myself at being negative about 50% of the time, I had a huge momentum shift in health and happiness.

24

Action steps to reduce anxiety and depression:
Easy:

Read *Spark: The Revolutionary New Science of Exercise and the Brain*, by John Ratey, MD. See your doctor to get approval to start half an hour of gentle aerobic and balancing exercises every day. Daily time spent walking has been shown to help anxiety and depression.

Anxiety and depression can also be caused by inflammation, nutritional deficiencies and lack of beneficial bacteria in our gut. Talk to an integrative, naturopathic or Ayurvedic doctor or nutritionist to get help.

Moderate:

With your doctor's okay, progress to high intensity aerobic exercise.

Read Donna Jackson Nakazawa's book *The Last Best Cure* for tips on walking meditation, among other things. Walking mindfully is incredibly calming, reducing both anxiety and depression.

Harder:

Read the book *Positive Psychology* by Martin Seligman. Take his online quiz at authentichappiness.org and see if you're as optimistic as you can be. If you catastrophize, try to stop the habit. You are keeping your unconscious paralyzed in fear. In the absence of confirmed knowledge, assume the best outcome—that's one way to start getting braver.

Develop your gratitude practice.

Take art classes, writing classes (be sure to journal, too), or music lessons to help activate the right brain. Use your non-dominant hand as much as possible to help develop your brain's less-used hemisphere. My lifelong anxiety began to turn around with daily journal writing and weekly meditation.

Chapter 3
Communicating with your Body

How the Brain Develops and How It Stays Healthy

We are born thinking with our entire brain. The way our brain interacts with the world is via the body moving and exploring. Babies react to stimuli with involuntary primary reflexes necessary to help them survive, such as sucking, swallowing, and hiccupping. Once each primitive reflex is mastered it gets handed off to the more primitive regions of the brain so that the cortex is free for higher thinking. Primary reflexes should not be present beyond a year of age, but can be reactivated or never properly inhibited when the baby experiences trauma or chronic stress. These reflexes can be reactivated in anyone by trauma at any age.

We want to have the most efficient use of each region of our brain. We do not want any part to be overused. The brain is harmed by having the more primitive areas over-activated by constant angry or fearful thoughts. Overuse of the sympathetic nervous system (also called SNS, our fight-or-flight system) creates an inflammatory body and brain state. The brain can also be harmed by not being fed correctly. Eating too much sugar or refined carbohydrates at one time can deprive the brain of fuel, triggering insulin production, which in turn causes cells to pull excess glucose out of the bloodstream and into fat storage.

Brain neurons are unable to store glucose so they rely on a steady source from our bloodstream. Hours after a coffee break or chocolatey afternoon snack, once the caffeine and sugar high wear off, insulin has caused blood sugar levels to crash. Most people will notice that they are feeling spacey, weak, confused or nervous. It is a signal that our brain has been harmed and that we have made poor nutritional choices.

The Vagus Nerve

The vagus nerve is the tenth cranial nerve. It supplies the parasympathetic motor connection for all the organs from the neck to the colon, except for the adrenal glands. The automatic processes of our bodies like heartbeat, breathing, blood pressure and body temperature are handled by our autonomic nervous system (ANS), which consists of the parasympathetic nervous system (PNS), the sympathetic nervous system (SNS), and our enteric nervous system (ENS). We need our PNS to be as strong as our SNS so that we can reset to calm after stress. The stronger our PNS is, the faster we return to calm after a stressful event. For those of us who have chronic stress, it usually means that the tone of our SNS is too high and our PNS has too low tone. I go into more details about developing the PNS in later chapters, but I also want to mention the PNS as being a central component to our social connection. Having low tone or having the myelinated part of the vagus nerve not sufficiently myelinated (as well as having other cranial nerves insufficiently myelinated) can reduce our ability to interact with others as well as decode nonverbal communication.

The information we receive from mirror neurons and non-verbal communication is processed by the right brain, which is another reason to make sure the right brain is fully developed.

In a study published by Psychological Science, the researchers, led by Barbara Frederickson and Bethany Kok found that people who experience warmer, more upbeat emotions may have better physical health because they make more social connections. The study also found that it is possible for a person to generate positive emotions for themselves using loving kindness meditation to make themselves physically healthier. Our vagus nerve also plays a role in satiation after eating. For these reasons, we want strong vagal tone.

The Importance of the Right Brain

The right brain oversees all unconscious processes, such as digestion, and our immune system. The more primitive areas of the brain are supposed to process vision if our primary reflexes have been properly mastered. When primary reflexes or gross motor skills (the ability to control the large muscles of the body for walking, running, sitting and crawling) are not properly developed or integrated, the cortex gets involved. Using the cortex this way diverts it from academic or creative thought. Instead, it is used to keep us physically safe by constantly checking our position as we interact with our environment.

The prefrontal cortex on the right side of the brain oversees the rhythm and timing in the body—things like our circadian rhythms, for example. as well as attention, and impulse control. Rhythm and timing are critical skills.

A lot of children, particularly boys, suffer from impulse control problems but the more active they are in rhythmic play like hopscotch, jump rope, bike riding, basketball, and soccer, the more this region of the brain gets developed and myelinated.

Being able to automatically process the information that a healthy vagus nerve provides is part of what keeps us from being on the autistic spectrum. Every autistic brain is different in what areas are underdeveloped and overdeveloped, but in general, information that can't be processed quickly enough is ignored, and not processing social information is a hallmark of autism. I think this is partly why so many children on the autistic spectrum benefit from a diet that eliminates gluten and dairy—if they're underdeveloped in processing speed, it's more likely their two hemispheres can't team properly to digest more difficult foods. A healthy vagus nerve keeps our digestion and immune system optimal too, as well as keeping us socially engaged and connected.

The parasympathetic nervous system is also involved in warming us up after a sudden exposure to cold. It's very popular in Finland and Russia to use a sauna to heat up, then go jump in the snow to cool off and start the cycle again. I believe they are giving their PNS a good workout. I would never recommend someone to try this who has an autoimmune disease. Start slow. People with poor vagal tone (which means low activity of the vagus nerve) have a great deal of difficulty warming up, particularly in winter time. I found it easier to start this process in the summer. I started with ice water splashed on my face (the vagus nerve runs through the face.) After I got used to that, I started working on increasing my tolerance for a shower with a cold-water blast. First, I take a warm shower, then I do a minute of cold water near the end. I particularly like this after a hot yoga session. I don't do it if I'm sick. People who are frustrated with having weak voices could likely use increased vagal tone, since it powers the larynx, pharynx and lungs. They could try adding in a bit of cold water exposure. I have more suggestions in the action steps at the end of this chapter.

The Steps Needed to Rebuild Health

If we find our health slipping, it is important to recognize the possible road to repair. What I have laid out are the most important things I've found to heal myself: flow, nutrition, internal repair, meditation, vision therapy, rhythm and timing therapies, left-brain healing therapies that have a right-brain connection, right-brain healing therapies, muscular/skeletal repair and muscle-based therapy relief.

I have examined what worked for me and what didn't. However, just because a therapy did not work well for me doesn't mean it won't work for you. I'll provide you with the information about what I have tried; you can choose what sounds best for you. We all have different comfort levels with left-brain and right-brain healing methods, so honor your needs and pick what your intuition tells you to try first.

If life takes an unexpected turn and your coping mechanisms aren't effective, I hope this book will be a resource for new ideas to regain your emotional, mental, spiritual or physical balance.

Action steps:
Easy:

Pay attention to your inner talk. When you feel anxious or depressed, look for the connection to the inner talk that caused it. Learning to notice these connections is a skill; it's the basis of starting the process of living your best life. Old thinking patterns slip in so quickly; they're automatic because they're what we've developed over the course of our life. Even one less negative thought about ourselves each day is a win.

Moderate:

Anxiety can be caused by histamine release. If you have lots of chronic stress, you may have leaky gut, and the histamine in your food could be causing anxiety and poor sleep. You might want to modify your diet. I go into more details in the Friday section of this book.

In addition to adding a minute of cold water at the end of a shower, or splashing the face in ice water, it's possible to increase vagal tone by doing the gentle breath-holding found in the meditation practice from Ligmincha that I teach. You can find out more about Ligmincha's inner and outer salung practice on my website, rightbrainuniversity.com, or take classes from them at ligmincha.org.

The vagus nerve can also be helped by things like humming and slow rhythmic breathing. As mentioned earlier, practicing loving-kindness meditation also increases tone. Remember, high vagal tone means your body can relax faster after being stressed. Low vagal tone means your body is likely stuck in chronic stress and unable to reset. I also found it helpful to gently add more social activity to help with vagal tone. It only works if you can find some type of social activity you don't mind, like volunteering for something that you enjoy, or if you're an introvert, going to the occasional party and helping out if you feel more comfortable that way. Be sure to honor when your body wants to leave.

Read more about the vagus nerve and how to help it in *The Self Hacked Secrets*, by Joseph Cohen.

Read Barbara Frederickson's book Love 2.0.

Harder:

Try Interactive Metronome (IM), which grows synaptic connections in the brain. Ask your IM trainer to focus on developing whichever hemisphere is weaker. In our culture, it's typically the right brain. Once that's done, have them integrate the left and right hemispheres. I'm an Interactive Metronome provider. You can find out more about Interactive Metronome and my work at Right Brain University in Chapter 19. You can find an IM trainer near you at interactivemetronome.com.

Monday:

Reduce Stress, Increase Flow

Chapter 4
Finding Flow

What is Flow?

Flow is any activity in which we become fully immersed in the experience, where we feel energized focus and enjoyment. You may know it as being 'in the zone.' Flow is a term coined by the positive psychology movement. What researchers found is that if we don't allow ourselves to experience flow, we suffer a deterioration of our mental health. In one study where participants were asked to stop immediately during the day each time they felt a sense of flow, the study had to be stopped after two days because of the participants' emotional state. Many of us who were raised by workaholics or authoritarians have a sense that if we are not producing something useful, it has no worth and therefore it isn't allowable. People like us feel guilty doing anything approaching play. It's taken a lot of doing the wrong thing (driving myself to get my novel completed is a good example) for me to learn that I have no choice about play. I need it and I am more productive if I get it. I'm also a lot happier and so is my family.

Any Activity Will Do

Being in a state of flow doesn't require we go out and buy art supplies. Each person is unique in what will create flow for them, and it can vary even within the same person from day to day. I get lost in flow when I am creating sculptures, writing, or walking on the beach. Some people find shopping at the supermarket to be incredibly stressful. I used to, but since completing vision therapy and Interactive Metronome treatment for ADHD (I'll go into detail in chapters 18 and 19), it's one of the highlights of my day if I am not overbooked. I've known people who find flow when they do the dishes, although I do not share this trait. I know others who find flow while driving a car. For years, driving required so much of my attention that it was anxiety-producing and exhausting. Vision therapy helped me so much that now I can find flow while driving too.

Even if we don't consider ourselves to be creative, it is essential that everyone have an outlet for flow. If we have no hobbies, no way to relax other than watching TV and the like, it's something we need to actively develop. Brené Brown, author of multiple books including *The Power of Vulnerability* saw the handwriting on the wall and started cultivating creativity after a lifetime of putting down artsy things like scrapbooking. It's now a favorite hobby of hers. Many of us were shamed as children by our teachers for our attempts to be creative in art, dance and writing. Once that happens, it becomes unsafe to be creative. We need to speak kindly to ourselves about our attempts at creativity.

Develop a Gratitude Practice

The positive psychology movement has given us tools to develop positivity and resilience. It's never too late—these skills can and should be learned by everyone. Positivity reduces our inner critic's activity and leads to resilience. I've found Martin Seligman's books *Authentic Happiness* and *Learned Optimism* as well as Mihaly Csikszentmihalyi's book *Flow: The Psychology of Optimal Experience* to be essential reading.

As I suggested before, you can take a free strengths survey at authentichappiness.org to help identify which skills to lean on and which skills need growing. I'd always considered myself an optimistic person, but the strengths survey helped me realize I had areas I could improve in. Doing so made me happier.

Above all, take the time to focus on things you are grateful for every day. I've read some suggestions to list three different things a day that you're grateful for and others that say to list five things a day. Start with three and work your way up if five seems unmanageable. Tuning your mind towards gratitude grows your time spent in calm and tells your unconscious that you value calm and joy. Stewing in how unhappy you are increases the stress in your life and will only add to your tendency to dwell on the negative. These are habits of thought. Do you want to develop a healthy habit or continue an unhealthy habit? You have the choice to change.

Start Journaling

Journaling is promoted to lower anxiety, stress and improve sleep. It's said to be a way to heal emotionally, physically and mentally, although I was skeptical of it. In case you are too, maybe you'll give it a try again after hearing how it's helped me. I have tried journaling multiple times, beginning in my childhood. I'd end up re-reading what I'd written a month or two later, judge it and rip it out. Whenever I find an old journal, the only thing left in it is a forlorn page or two. I learned what journaling can do for a person after I turned forty. Journaling regularly is an opportunity to become your own best friend, to be able to figure out how you feel about something, and to experience saying anything and being loved no matter what. Once I finally understood this lesson, it helped me begin to thrive. Often, we don't know how we feel until we talk about what's happening in our lives. It's getting rarer that we have enough people in our lives who can bear hearing everything that we need to express. We move a lot, which can disrupt friendships. It's said that our electronic devices are making us less connected too. It's good practice to connect with one's gut and learn how to be positive and encouraging to oneself. There are a lot of daily complaints and stressors that come up in journaling, but that once we release that, there's a lot of time spent noticing the intricacy and beauty of life. I find that gets overlooked if I'm not journaling and practicing gratitude.

Writing to Heal

Writing to heal is also valuable and helps the left and right brain to understand and assimilate traumatic events in our lives. If you took the ACE test that I mentioned earlier (the test is in the Appendix), you'll have a sense if you need writing to heal. I encourage everyone to try it. Life is hard for all of us; even the luckiest of us were helpless children at some point. Understanding how to reframe scary events so that we can see how we learned important lessons from them is something that leads us to personal growth and healing. It allows the right and left hemispheres of the brain to begin operating on the same frequency. When we block the memory consciously in the left brain, the right brain is still reliving it under the radar. This way both hemispheres can go forward together. If you are interested in writing a book, both journaling and writing to heal provide a wealth of emotional material for developing one. It's important to let what you've written settle for some number of months to lose its emotional charge before using it for fiction work. I let mine sit for five months minimum.

Behavioral Epigenetics

Behavioral epigenetics is a study of cellular traits that change because of external or environmental factors. These factors can change not just in ourselves, but can be passed along through multiple generations without changing the DNA. A study with mice at Emory University showed that fear of the smell of cherry blossoms (which was paired with a shock to the foot) is inheritable through two generations. It's very likely that humans are impacted by this, but we've got a heck of a lot more brain than mice do, so it could impact many more generations. If so, that makes it even more important to learn to process trauma so that future generations won't be affected. One of the biggest environmental factors we can change is how we think about ourselves, how patient we are with ourselves, and whether we shame ourselves for making mistakes. These thoughts create toxic changes in our bodies at a cellular level and yet we do it anyway. We wrongly assume being supportive of ourselves will cause an inflated ego. I am not suggesting that we do this in a narcissistic way, but rather like a loving parent or coach would. When we allow constant negativity towards ourselves, essentially we are providing our own shock to the foot. Please understand I'm not talking about a free-for-all/anything-goes type of scenario. There's a middle ground. For too long, I was strongly in the toxic shame camp without understanding what I was doing to myself. It's taken me a long time to learn how to live in balance.

The Power of Nitric Oxide

In her book *"Goddesses Never Age,"* Christianne Northrup speaks of the power of nitric oxide, which is released in peak experience such as pleasure, creativity or orgasm. We want to make sure we have a peak experience of some kind every day. This is the flow that positive psychologists are talking about. To produce nitric oxide, we must have sufficient vitamin D. We also must allow ourselves the time to be unproductive, to get away from what "must" be done and have some play time, no matter what our to-do lists say. I speak as a recovering perfectionist and a recovering workaholic. It's still a challenge despite all I've learned to make sure I take an entire day off once a week. It's a challenge to build in flow/peak experiences every day. I'm also much lower in vitamin D than I should be, as are most Americans. Rebuilding that level has been a top priority of mine. I want to support my body's ability to produce nitric oxide. I make sure to take vitamin D with vitamin K to avoid tissue calcification.

Action steps:
Easy:
Take the time to identify what puts you into a flow state and think about how to add it to your life regularly.

Pick up a fresh piece of paper and a crayon every day and scribble something on it. Pay attention to how you feel as you do it, and also as you pat yourself the back for what you did. If you're uncomfortable doing childish things like patting yourself on the back, try to grow your tolerance for it.

If you love art, do a little every day.

Start journaling.

Start a gratitude practice.

Try writing to heal. Dr. James Pennebaker's book *Writing to Heal* is a great place to start learning how.

Moderate:

Take a class in something creative that you always wanted to do some day—-and make it a weekly priority to practice it.

Reading uplifting books or shows can put us in a flow state. I enjoy watching Oprah's *Super Soul Sunday* interviews on oprah.com.

I also like Jack Canfield's *Chicken Soup for the Soul* series, along with Marci Shimoff's book *Happy for No Reason.* Think about what lifts you up and do more of that.

Meditation can put you into a flow state. Try Oprah and Deepak Chopra's free 21 Day meditation programs, which are wonderful.

Monitor self-talk in a loving way.

Harder:

Ask your doctor if you should get your vitamin D levels checked and prescribed a supplement if you're low.

Chapter 5
Meditation 101

I'd always been a meditation avoider—I'd tried it during yoga classes I'd gone to back in the late 1990's and hated it because it made me more anxious as well as increasing my anxiety and ADHD symptoms. I would be calm from doing yoga only to find myself agitated by the meditation. It made me feel like there was something wrong with me. Fortunately, in 2006 I found a form of Tibetan Bön/Buddhist Tsa-Lung meditation that worked for me, which I now teach. Bön combines meditation with movement and breath exercises that allow the body to calm down enough so that the mind can finally get quiet.

Why we should Meditate

Meditation helps increase our ability to concentrate because it gives us practice in concentrating. It does not matter whether you succeed in having fewer thoughts or no thoughts. It is the repeated attempts to observe our thoughts that helps develop the ability to be mindful.

Meditation helps protect against aging as it builds additional grey matter in our brain, so our brain stays younger longer. It improves our ability not to be swept along by our emotions because we learn to observe ourselves and our thoughts. It also helps us to remain in our highest level of thinking, executive thought, rather than triggered into reacting with our emotional or primitive brain.

The Benefits of Observing Ourselves

With practice, we will be able to observe ourselves, our thoughts and emotions and stay centered as higher levels of thinking stay active. Many of us pay attention to thoughts or feelings as being of primary importance in directing our lives. We think our thoughts and feelings are always right and should be acted upon. With regular practice, we can eventually realize that while it's important to honor and process our emotions, it is not good to act on them without rational reflection. Meditation allows us to access our prefrontal cortex so we can have that rational review. It allows us to be better at our jobs and in our relationships. Our thoughts and emotions are a constantly changing landscape. If we think of our right brain as a vast blue sky (since the non-judgment of the right brain is always peaceful and calm) and the left brain's anxiety and anger as storm clouds, we can see why it might be better to attempt to focus on the calming vastness of the clear blue sky than it is on the grey storm clouds of emotion and thought. The sky is always there, even if we can't see it. We can access it through meditation. The calm of the non-judgmental right brain is connected to our intention even when our left brain is ready to give up and act out. We can stay on a more even keel, a more level path, if we meditate.

Four Types of Meditation

Being able to remain calmer lowers stress and increases health by reducing use of the sympathetic nervous system's (SNS) inflammatory pathway. Once I mastered Tibetan Bön meditation, other types of meditation opened up for me. The five types of meditation that have been most helpful to me are:

1) Bön meditation, a type of Tibetan meditation, uses movement and breath-holding to calm the nervous system enough to allow stillness without panic, even for ADHD types like me. It changed my life. It's hard to explain, but easily followed. You can find YouTube links by searching for videos by Ligmincha, an institute founded by my teacher's teacher Wangyal Tenzin Rinpoche. They

have three main practices that I've enjoyed: the Outer Tsa-Lung, Inner Tsa-Lung and Secret Tsa-Lung. (Contact info for all five types is at the end of this chapter.)

2) Vipasana meditation at its simplest uses the basics of thinking, "Rising" on an *in* breath and "Falling" on an *out* breath. It's normal to constantly be distracted and start thinking and feeling again. When we do, simply return to thinking, "Rising" on an *in* breath and "Falling" on an *out* breath. We can't get it wrong, it's all about eventually remembering to think "Rising" and "Falling." Some days my mind is so busy that I don't remember until a minute before the timer goes off at the end of the session—but there's no blame or shame because I've gotten my practice in by trying.

3) Open Focus meditation is proven to produce alpha waves (that's good) and reset the hypothalamic axis stress response (that's good too.) The shortest version of their meditation practice is only seven minutes long. I've found longer versions to be helpful in reducing pain as well as calming me. The idea is to focus on the space between things rather than focusing on objects.

4) Oprah and Deepak Chopra's meditation programs.

5) TAT meditation, created by John Douillard, gives multiple meditative tools using breathing. It's more to learn, but I've found it's always good in a crisis to have lots of tools to choose from.

Meditation and Impermanence of Emotions

Meditation is helpful for learning that feelings are impermanent. This was a revelation to me; I thought that bad feelings hung around, waiting to strike when least expected.

I learned this in 2006, when every Monday I attended a writing class at the Hudson Valley Writer's Center and every Tuesday I took a meditation class. My meditation teacher, Annegret Wolfe Rice, was trained at Ligmincha by Tenzin Wangyal Rinpoche. Annegret led us through meditation, readings and recordings from his books *Tibetan Sound Healing,* as well as *Healing with Form, Energy and Light.*

Every week as I journaled and wrote, emotions came up that could have blocked me. But thanks to the meditation, I realized that I could feel utterly horrible at the start of a meditation practice and feel transformed and peaceful within a half an hour of practice. That changed my whole outlook on fear and anxiety. For my entire life, I had avoided doing anything that might scare me because I was so terrified of the feelings that would come up. But now I realized I didn't have to be limited in that way anymore.

I realized that my emotions weren't necessarily right. A lot of what I experienced as fear, anger or anxiety was because my primitive brain was hijacking my mind and taking over my thinking process. That then generated a flood of potentially incorrect conclusions and emotions. I realized meditation was important to get to a state of calm and to not make decisions based on my primitive and emotional brain's thinking.

Action steps:
Easy:

Try to focus on your breath every day when you wake up, go to sleep or get upset. This is a way to train yourself to stay in the moment. If you get upset, focus on breath rather than the volatility of your emotions. This can help calm you down. Over time, this creates a new habitual reaction.

Moderate:

Practice Bon, TAT or Open Focus by taking part in a once-a-week class. More on Bön at ligmincha.org, Oprah and Deepak Chopra's at chopra.com. TAT at lifespa.com, and Open Focus at openfocus.com.

Harder:

Bring your practice into daily life. Go on a meditation retreat. Join me for one of mine. More info at rightbrainuniversity.com.

Chapter 6
Give Yoga or Dance a Try

Yoga still seems so foreign and strange to many people in America. Lots of people try it, but many don't stick with it because it's too different or appears to have too much of a learning curve. One way to get at the unprocessed emotions that are lodged in our bodies is through yoga, so it's worth the effort to develop a yoga practice.

Yoga has the potential to help or harm us. It can help us if we begin to connect to our bodies and start listening to what the body wants. Our body is our guide, so we must surrender our egos when we walk in the door. Yoga will grow our attention span for checking in with the body. If a pose feels hard to do, modify it. Keep checking in with the body. It will be hard to do at first. At some point, newcomers will notice that they've checked out. That's when they can bring their attention back to feeling into the body. There is no shame at checking out and going on autopilot. We just want to start shifting into being present. The more we practice this, the better we get at it. This is one of the main benefits of yoga, this close connection to our body. Mostly we ignore the body until it hurts. We can take what we learn on the mat out into our daily lives and improve our ability to heal and be centered in the present moment.

If we don't work at increasing that connection, it's easy to overstretch. That's how yoga can harm us. Competing with other people to do or outdo what they're doing on their mat is the perfect way to get hurt.

Learning from our Emotions

Our bodies are constantly trying to get us to learn from our emotions. To understand this through a blend of chiropractic and Traditional Chinese Medicine, the idea is that neuropeptides for the same emotion are sent to the same regions of the body along the same meridian pathway.

Whenever something happens to us which is like something that happened to us before, the same muscles are activated as in the original incident, reactivating an old unprocessed emotion. The stretching in yoga allows for opportunity to process, learn and release these emotions.

People who have negative associations to yoga might have sensed that uncomfortable emotions were coming up. Our primitive brain is scared of emotions, so we may reject yoga in order to make our primitive brain more comfortable.

It can take a lot of grit to start a yoga practice knowing that we might be emotionally uncomfortable, but the explanation of why it feels uncomfortable can encourage us all to stick it out. Over time, we'll release toxic, inflammatory neurochemicals, something we don't want in our bodies. Our health is too important.

Svaroopa Yoga

The easiest yoga I've ever tried is Svaroopa, a type of restorative yoga that is so comfortable and relaxing that I call it "Couch Potato Yoga." Instructors are trained to be aware of an individual's body alignment so they can put us into the proper position to allow our bodies to relax.

In Svaroopa it is believed when the hips, shoulder blades and head are perfectly aligned and flat while laying on a comfortable blanket, the body can begin to release tension; it sure worked for me. I had a much higher level of muscle tension when I first started doing Svaroopa yoga and nothing came close to reducing muscle tension so directly, particularly in my head and shoulders. No other restorative yoga classes have ever done as much for me. While it's very easy, it's also profound in its ability to release. After the first class, it felt like I was coming down with the flu, only it consisted of aches of sadness and other emotions rather than the usual flu aches as these neurochemicals were released. I never experienced discomfort again after the first two classes, only deep comfort and relaxation. I recommend drinking plenty of water to help process the neurochemicals that get released.

You can often get a lot from a yoga class at private studios in your home town or at your local YMCA. Just keep trying out different styles of yoga until you find one that works for you, along with an encouraging teacher and friendly class vibe.

Russayog

One unique form of yoga is called Russayog, which has pop-up classes in Santa Barbara, as well as DVDs available online. It can provide as much or as little of a workout as you want. Their yoga practice combines yoga with ropes to help provide stability for people who are uncomfortable with their ability to balance. It also provides innovative movements which harness positivity in the body. The body responds to movement in a way that many of us don't understand--for example, holding our arms overhead in a v-shape generates a more positive mental state, while holding arms below the waist generates a more downcast state. This is something I learned from a Waldorf School's Eurythmy dance instructor, so I look for elements of that wherever I can find it. Russayog's warmup and cool-down hand and arm movements leave me uplifted.

Hot Yoga

I've gotten a lot of help from hot yoga. In 2011, while on a writers' retreat on Martha's Vineyard, I had an osteopathic physician-in-training, Andy Estrella, tell me my spine was near the point of no return from degeneration. He recommended Bikram Yoga to help me bring it back. At that point, 90 minutes of hot yoga sounded like a joke: I had chronic fatigue and fibromyalgia and have always loathed being too hot. But I was desperate enough to try it because I'd had some spinal stenosis symptoms. After three months of Bikram in 2011, normal sensation returned. I've stuck with hot yoga ever since.

Most of the people I've met with Fibromyalgia do not exercise. They feel like they can't; they are too tired. I totally understand that because I went through that, too. I found that my anxiety and ADHD symptoms worsened whenever I gave in to listening to how tired I felt. I hated feeling anxious more than I hated feeling tired, so I continued to try to exercise. It was very hard, but I always felt better for having done it. Even at times when I was at my worst levels of pain, anxiety and depression, I would have these brief windows where I would feel normal from having gone to hot yoga, so I knew I was doing the right thing.

Putting up with Short-Term Humiliation for Long-Term Rewards

Because of the chronic fatigue, I've spent more time on my back in a hot yoga class than most people ever spend in a yoga studio in their entire lives. At first, I went once a week and it took me about four hours to recover from class. But I felt normal for about half an hour later that first day, for the first time in eight years, so I was hooked. Once I could stay upright for an entire class, I then moved on to adding a second class per week. Once I could stay upright for both classes a week, I moved on to three classes a week. Three years ago, I switched to Core Power, a national hot yoga chain. I love it because classes are only an hour long and the teachers are kind and encouraging. I have more time for my day and find the class length to be perfect for energizing me.

I've also stuck with hot yoga because sweating is a good way to rid the body of toxins—autoimmune illness causes the body to accumulate toxins--and I want to support their release.

The Benefits of Dance

Dance classes can also get our emotions moving and releasing. Unfortunately, many people are self-critical when it comes to their ability to dance, but if you can be a good coach to yourself, you can enjoy dance no matter your current skill level. If you consider yourself too uncoordinated, be sure to read about Vision Therapy in Chapter 18, since even people with perfect vision can need prism glasses to enable them to see 3-D.

Dance helps the brain to integrate itself. Moving forward, backward, up, down, jumping, spinning around are all things that make the two hemispheres of the brain talk to each other and become better coordinated. Most towns offer lots of different types of dance to choose from, so try out whatever your town has available. Consider your local YMCA, recreation center and private studios, depending on your budget. In Santa Barbara, we are blessed to have an amazing Zumba teacher, Josette Tkacik, who has used Zumba as part of a program to heal herself from Advanced Rheumatoid Arthritis. Every day between 150-300 people attend her class, where she teaches about the importance of finding and following your passion, knowing you are here for a purpose, and living in non-judgment, all while delivering a terrific workout. People (yes, women and men) of all ages and abilities come together to share the joy of movement and community.

Bhangra Dance

If you're open to multi-cultural types of dance, the husband-wife team behind Russayog, Jasprit and Teresa Singh, who are always looking to help people develop a healthier mind-body lifestyle, have created Bhangra Dance, which is available online.

Histamine

If you have unexplained weakness at times, going from feeling strong to feeling weak and exhausted, it's possible that the immune system is dealing with histamine sensitivity or mast cell activation.

Exercise can activate histamine and mast cells. Be sure to pay close attention when reading the Friday section of this book. It turned out to be a huge help for me in my energy levels.

Action steps:
Easy:

If you're healthy, get your doctor's okay to try something simple like Svaroopa or another type of restorative yoga class.

Tune into how you're talking to yourself before a class, so that you are kind and encouraging. Be patient; reset your thinking in a positive, loving way before each class. I loved my Svaroopa teacher in NY, Sue Kessman-Krieger, who can be reached at suekk1@verizon.net.

You can learn about Russayog Yoga and Bhangra Dance through their YouTube Channel *Russayog Yoga*. DVDs are available at yogadancepower.com.

Find a dance dvd or youtube video you like. One funny, upbeat YouTube video series is The Fitness Marshall. He pairs hit songs with hip-hop moves and explains everything well. If you think you need to be thin to dance, think again, because one of his dancers is large-sized and inspirational in her fitness level and dance ability. Just get your doctor's okay before trying it.

Moderate:

Try a more active yoga class. Yoga styles vary from more constant movement to more static holds. Find something that feels comfortable for you with encouraging teachers. Avoid classes where teachers judge you or tell you to move in a way that feels unsafe. That's not real yoga.

You can find out more information about Josette, Santa Barbara's premier Zumba teacher, at josettetkacik.com.

Harder:

If you struggle with your health and have your doctor's blessing to try hot yoga, look for a studio near you. Heat can make us overstretch without realizing it, so monitor yourself and don't go too far your first few classes. Our bodies have developed fascia (discussed more in the next chapter) over the course of our lifetime to protect us, so tread cautiously. If you are not careful, you can go beyond what your body is ready for, which can either lead to injury or alarm in your body. Honor your body by being gentle with yourself. Go slow, drink plenty of water and lie down as often as needed.

Core Power has locations across the country. You can find them online at corepoweryoga.com. They offer unheated and moderately heated yoga classes too. If you're interested in CPY, get your doctor's okay first. I'd suggest starting with their unheated classes and work your way into heated.

Chapter 7
Trying RSFT

Most of us have not heard of Resistance Flexibility Strength Training (RFST) before, despite it being featured as Oprah's exercise of choice in the January 2016 issue of "O Magazine." It's like yoga, only more profound in its ability to change us quickly. I think it's an easier practice to get into as well. The trainers I've met make a point of trying to make it accessible to people who haven't exercised in years.

RFST has centers in Boston and Santa Barbara, as well as trainers in Los Angeles and New York. If you're not near these cities, you can benefit from buying Bob Cooley's new book "*Resistance Flexibility 1.0: Becoming Flexible in All Ways*," or by trying their online training videos at geniusofflexibility.com.

It's All About the Fascia

Bob Cooley began developing RFST in the 1970's after trying to recover from a devastating automobile accident. He had recovered from many of his physical injuries, but something was still very wrong. Only stretching with resistance made a difference to his health. In researching why, he learned about fascia, a network of tissue which attaches muscle to bone, skin to muscle, and surrounds our organs. Fascia is an instantaneous neural feedback network, but it can become dense and overgrown from physical injury as well as excess thinking or emotion. It's possible to break up the excess fascia and when you do, it feels wonderful, joyful, invigorating, and liberating. The best news is that there is no pain from breaking up dense fascia because it doesn't have nerve attachments to it.

Why we Have Dense Fascia

People with constant stress or who have had physical injuries from sports or auto accidents will have lots of dense fascia in their bodies. We accept these limitations because no one's taught us any differently. Bob's done enough research experimenting on himself to learn that dense fascia can impair the function of our internal and external immune systems. It can also impair our endocrine system and more, which can lead to pain and constriction, which can in turn impair our thought patterns and emotions.

Stretching under resistance contracts the muscle while the fascia resists, which helps reorient it and break it down. Breaking down dense fascia permanently changes it. We can re-grow it, but the practice of resistance stretching can help improve our thought patterns, which makes it less likely that we'd regrow the same amount of dense fascia. Other treatments such as chiropractic can give us immediate relief, but then our patterns of fascia generated from thoughts or emotional tension can shift our bones out of alignment again.

Our Dominant and Weakest Meridians

Bob also realized that our genetic profiles and our childhoods impact us as to which meridians are dominant and which are our weakest links. This helps to bring awareness to our way of interacting with the world. We all have patterns of interacting with the world: some of us do so in a thinking way, some of us in a feeling way, some of us in a spiritual way, some of us in a physical way. It can make it hard to understand other people when our experience of the world is so different. Doing resistance stretching allows us to integrate these different types of patterns into our minds and bodies so that we can be more whole and complete.

Attending trainings has helped me understand others'

differences and appreciate them for what they've been through. I've heard many others in class say the same thing. They find it easier to be in the world. They notice how much happier, how much more physically comfortable, and how much more connected they are to their family and people in their community. I think it's especially good for thinking types as compared to some of the other techniques I have tried. Thinking types notice that they have less pain and more flexibility. As a result, they become more whole, rather than just being in their heads all the time.

Weekly Classes and Weekend Trainings

RFST centers offer weekly classes, as well as weekend trainings that I'd highly recommend. I've attended RFST's levels 1-3, taught by the talented Elite Trainer duo Luther Cowden and Nick Ware. At each level, I felt a sense of increasing freedom. Instead of being held prisoner in a straightjacket of fascia, I had more range of motion, a lighter body and lighter, faster thoughts. Should this sound a bit too strenuous for your level of fitness, there's a gentle type of fascia stretching called John Barnes Myofascial Release technique (MFR.) I'll go into this later in Chapter 11.

Action steps:
Easy:

If you're well, I'd recommend the book *Resistance Flexibility 1.0* to help you develop a regular stretching routine. Streaming videos are available online at geniusofflexibility.com if you need further guidance.

Moderate:

If your health could use improving, I'd recommend attending a class or a weekend training program. Many who try it switch to RFST as their stretching program of choice, giving up their yoga practice as unnecessary, however I love my hot yoga too much to give it up.

Harder:

Begin working with a trainer. There's so much that RFST trainers can do to give you back the healthy body you were born with. Bob still works directly with clients, as do Luther Cowden and Nick Ware. I've done weekly sessions in Santa Barbara with trainers Samuel Camburn, Red, and Richard Gregston, which have helped reset incorrect patterns of movement. The centers are filled with a wonderful staff of enthusiastic trainers. I've also done a fibromyalgia-specific intensive with Luca Cupery and Kaj Hoffman who received special training from Bob to help those with fibromyalgia. It's quickly brought me to new levels of energy I haven't seen since before my auto accident. A friend of mine with ME/CFS, formerly known as chronic fatigue syndrome, has been getting a lot of help through RFST with her trainer Karen Mason in Santa Barbara, who also received special pointers from Bob to help target ME/CFS.

Tuesday:

Understand Pain

Chapter 8
Pain and Its Message

My Pain History

I had stomach pain growing up since I was about seven or eight. I thought it was normal. I slept poorly for most of my life and thought it was never going to change. My body, especially my neck and shoulder, hurt since not long after I broke my collarbone at age seven. After a whiplash car accident when I was thirty-nine, my chronic shoulder and neck pain grew much worse and I started developing numbness, tingling and difficulty walking, as well as worsening bouts of stomach pain and IBS attacks. Neurologists ruled out multiple sclerosis, but it took me years to finally get a diagnosis of fibromyalgia.

Fibromyalgia Pain

Doctors now know that the pain of fibromyalgia is due to extremely excessive amounts of a type of nerve fiber called arteriole-venule (AV) shunts. They are talking about developing treatments based on this type of nerve fiber. I have a good friend with Cerebral Palsy, who says that by the age of forty, most CP patients also develop fibromyalgia. Since CP patients tend to suffer a great many falls over the course of their lives, it seems possible that excessive amounts of AV shunts occur because of physical trauma as opposed to a purely genetic cause, particularly because many CP patients develop CP because of birth trauma rather than a genetic link. This ties into the onset of many non-CP patients with fibromyalgia—onset happened after a whiplash car accident or multiple falls. I mention all of this because most people with fibromyalgia have been treated like our problems are imaginary, when really, medicine hadn't advanced enough to know what was wrong. Thank goodness for progress.

Much of our Pain is Hidden from us by our Autonomic Nervous System

A lot of pain is hidden by the brain via endorphins, oxytocin and dopamine; this means we frequently do not get a direct sense of cause and effect. We often don't become aware of pain until it reaches the point at which it can no longer be suppressed. Emotional pain becomes physical pain. Mental over-thinking can become physical pain. Our physical pain can become emotional and mental pain. It all runs on the same circuit board. A healthy brain produces enough endorphins so that the connection between emotional, mental and physical pain is hidden as we go about in our daily lives. This is a hidden form of fight-or-flight that we are living with. Years of holding onto emotions and thoughts build up until our bodies are toxic. Once we no longer have healthy levels of endorphins, the pain becomes constant. Physical pain can become emotional and mental pain as our physical state leads to depression or sadness or anger at our physical limitations or degeneration. We can get caught up in over-thinking as we try to figure a way out of the situation. As a result, another round of emotional and mental pain also gets stored in the body, adding to our pain and risk of disease as inflammatory neurochemicals continue to build up.

Picking up Other People's Emotional States

I've learned that my pain levels are worse if I'm around other people who are in a painful emotional state. Our mirror neurons can pick up other people's energy and hold it within us. That's a normal human reaction, but most people aren't aware of it because it's processed unconsciously. Our pain gets taken on by others in the same way—that's why it can sometimes feel so hard to be around people who are in emotional pain. Our healing lessens the load on others, as their mirror neurons pick up on our healed state and hold that healthy energy. We can then become a catalyst for change and healing in other people.

Understanding this is why I took on the task of fully healing. I want to live as healthily as I can for as long as I'm alive on this good earth, be an example for my children, as well as a catalyst for healing in others.

Sleep Quality is Essential

Sleep quality, soundness of sleep and the amount of Rapid Eye Movement (REM) cycle time is essential for keeping levels of pain at their lowest. REM cycle is the deep sleep we are in when we dream, typically 90-120 minutes per night. Chronic stress and nutritional deficiencies can impact our ability to sleep soundly which can then set off an inflammatory cycle in our brain and body.

Pain is stored in Muscle Memory

I believe that pain is stored in muscle memory as tension. The emotion felt at the time of the injury also gets stored. Much of our physical pain is accumulated emotional pain. Much of our emotional pain is due to stewing over our thoughts. Since emotional pain gets stored in our bodies, our thoughts create physical pain too.

Judging thoughts about others and their actions create tension within us. And our judging thoughts about our own actions can lead to bad moods and a domino effect of further bad actions. It negatively impacts our own internal climate, family life and time with friends. I think we humans are basically judgment machines because judging is a basic survival mechanism. I've found that I feel better the less I judge others. It's a way of reducing my internal stress, because our unconscious does not understand the difference between us and other. Our unconscious hides parts of ourselves from our conscious awareness to protect us. When we were young children, anytime our parents or society rejected our behavior in a traumatic way, our unconscious hid that part away. When we judge another person, our unconscious knows that there is a part of us that is or was a little bit like that person. It causes stress for our unconscious and leads to dissociation, which is a lack of conscious connection to our thoughts or emotions. They get hidden from our conscious awareness by our unconscious in order to protect us. Debbie Ford's book, *The Dark Side of the Light Chasers,* has a more detailed explanation.

Becoming Aware of When We are Under Stress

It's important to become more aware of our stressed states, so that when we are causing our own stress we can learn to let it go.

Have you ever lost or forgotten something that made you upset? Can you remember what you thought about yourself? Can you remember if you were kind?

Most of us have a usual pattern of getting down on ourselves for forgetting or losing something. We internally beat ourselves up for forgetting and berate ourselves to never forget again. Maybe there's a possibility of finding it, so we start stewing about the likelihood of it getting stolen before we can retrace our steps or contact someone to check if they'd found it.

How Self-Judging Hurts our Loved Ones

When we started beating ourselves up internally, it makes us feel bad about ourselves and that creates internal tension which always (despite our best intentions) gets taken out on other people. Who are we around most? Our family and friends. Who will be the bearer of our tension? Our family and friends. Because we've made them suffer, they will have higher stress levels, which will bounce back to us.

Next time you forget something, try using it as an opportunity for personal growth. When I turn around and forgive myself for forgetting and let all my expectations go, I relax, enjoy the day, feel happy and smile way more than usual. I enjoy the beauty of the people that I come across, all because of being loving and kind toward myself. I feel so happy, all of me, my unconscious and my conscious. I feel grateful for eventually remembering what I'd forgotten so I can try to retrieve it. I give thanks for what I have in my life and for the fact that I usually have a very good memory. All of this reduces my internal tension, which means less tension for my family and friends. Why would I live any other way? It just doesn't make sense, does it?

And yet so many people have the same pattern of beating the tar out of their inner selves in this way for making mistakes. The stats are that 3,999 people out of 4,000 want to please others; that is the ratio of normal people to sociopaths.

We are Parenting Ourselves Our Whole Life

Our unconscious wants to please us. We are the parent of our unconscious self for the rest of our life. Be a good one. Knowing that I am my own parent is a game changer for the quality of my life. I have found that making someone else "pay" for how they've treated me only generates long term harm for myself.

No matter how much someone else loves me, they are not going to be obsessing about how much harm or injustice they caused me. Either they feel bad and resolve to do better or they don't. Either way they end up moving on.

Meanwhile I have created a toxic environment in my body because of obsessing over the situation. Far better to process how I feel and either move on from the relationship or realize that someone else might have reacted differently to the same situation. Other people don't "make" me feel anything— my own unique history and neural pathways, plus the type of day I'm having all combine to generate my feelings. Same thing holds true for other human beings.

Interactions with Other People are a Mirror for Us to see Our Own "Stuff"

Seeing the same kind of emotions recur time after time in our life is a mirror for us to realize that we have anger (or whatever other emotion is coming up) that needs to be worked through. We might react in anger at all the many angry people we come across, not understanding that other people might react with compassion to the same situation. I believe that we all have default programming that we are put here to learn how to rise above when we are triggered.

Not being true to oneself puts one into pain, contraction, and inflammation. This is because of the increased primitive brain and emotional brain activation. If, for example, someone stays in a relationship out of fear of the unknown, it means they are ignoring the emotional information from the unhappiness they feel that their needs aren't being met, rather than using their unhappiness as an opportunity to grow. Meanwhile, that unhappiness is causing pain, contraction and inflammation that can lead to disease. So is living with fear of the unknown rather than learning how to take steps to stop being frozen by fear in their lives.

Changing Our Response to Pain

I am all for working things out in relationships, but a clear-eyed view of a situation is also helpful. How can we become our best self in a way that might inspire others to be their best selves? How can we become our best self unless we learn to be kind to ourselves? I've realized that just because we have physical, mental and emotional pain does not mean that we should allow ourselves to be immobilized by the pain or the fear of pain. When I was under emotional or mental tension, I needed to find a way to release the tension from my body. That tension was a wakeup call that something wasn't working in my life and needed to be addressed. Taking pain seriously as an indication of stress is an important part of the process.

Some people let go of outcomes and pray for help, which I believe really works. At a minimum, I suspect it activates something in the unconscious that takes pressure away from the ego self.

Action steps:
Easy:

Realize that thinking kind thoughts about yourself and redirecting negative or judging thoughts about others will help reduce contraction and pain in your body. Self-compassion was the biggest healer for me when I was depressed. Through self-compassion, I found the motivation and ability to act.

Try prayer. Even if you're an atheist or agnostic, try praying to the collective unconscious or to the unknown capacities of the human mind and heart. There is far more to our brains' abilities than science yet understands, and as I said before, I think it reduces pressure on our unconscious. For those who are not depressed, try the moderate or harder action steps below:

Moderate:

Try Open Focus meditation, developed by Les Fehmi, at openfocus.com. Open Focus meditation helps produce alpha waves in the brain and can reset the stress axis that keeps us in fight or flight mode. It helps us focus on the space between things, rather than on the objects we see around us. Taking in visual data and processing it into objects is a contractive process. This is because it can overuse our focal vision system, which activates our fight-or-flight sympathetic nervous system. Over time, constant contraction adds up to pain.

Harder:

Begin a program using RFST's book *Resistance Flexibility 1.0,* which helps release and realign the body where injury, thought and emotion have caused fascia growth and contraction. Some of RFST's online videos (available at thegeniusofflexibility.com) are specifically geared to stop neck or other specific pain.

Try hot yoga or another form of yoga that you connect with. Most hot yoga studios offer cooler or unheated classes for beginners.

Try cognitive hypnotherapy to reduce conditioned responses to life's stresses.

Chapter 9
Musculo-skeletal Repair

After decades of high tension, my body started to break down. Here's what I've discovered that helped:

Physical Therapy

I learned the hard way to get multiple recommendations for a physical therapist. Even so, I've found a difference going to a physical therapist who has a PhD. I broke my collarbone when I was seven and despite going to physical therapists off and on for help over the years, no one figured out that my arm was out of the socket because of that broken bone. It only took my PhD therapist back in New York two visits to realize why I had chronic shoulder and neck pain. There are plenty of wonderful physical therapists without a PhD. My current PT in California doesn't have one. Get your recommendations and if you don't feel better after treatment, move on to a new person. Try searching out someone with a PhD if you can't get relief.

Physical therapy helps to release muscle tension, increase strength, and educate clients about what is wrong with how we use our bodies. It works best when combined with a whole-body exercise like swimming, yoga or RFST, so that all the muscles get strengthened.

Chiropractic

From what I've read, medical researchers now think of

meridians as nerve and fascia highways. Chiropractors think of meridian pathways as nerve pathways. I've gotten a lot of pain relief and increased mobility from going to a chiropractor. Their work corrects spinal alignment to allow for proper nerve flow. But why does the spine get out of alignment? Very likely because of dense fascia. Why does fascia shift our bones? Because of trauma, whether physical, mental or emotional. Ultimately, we can have back problems because of mental and emotional issues too, not just physical injury. Our back muscles contract when we have a feeling of danger or the urge to move away from something. They ease up when we have a feeling of safety or desire to move towards something or connect with it. Over time, constantly feeling in danger (chronic stress telling our bodies that we are unsafe) keeps our muscles contracted until we are locked into spasm. Again, I find it important to combine chiropractic with RFST or John Barnes MFR to break up or rearrange old fascia, as well as release emotional patterns.

The most helpful chiropractors I've been to combine nutrition with balancing the nervous system. I wouldn't be without a good chiropractor, but I make sure that I work on processing my thoughts and feelings, so that I'm not expecting my chiropractor to do all the work without any help from me. Occasionally I go to my chiropractor, get adjusted and my back immediately goes out again. I can always trace it to a thought or emotion that I was having. I've learned not to lock into fear around it. I find it almost always goes away within a few minutes if I use the ESR/K27 diagram in Chapter 15 while providing myself a supportive thought to replace the stressful one. If that ever happens to you, see if this combination helps you reset your spine too.

Osteopathic Physician's Cranial Sacral Therapy

I've found Cranial Sacral Therapy as done by an osteopathic physician to be of enormous help. The muscles contract in a way that can prevent proper flow of spinal fluid from the cranium to the sacrum and osteopaths can get things flowing again. My osteopath's suggestion of trying Bikram yoga to help reduce spinal stenosis symptoms was genius; it helped change my patterns of using my body. Remember that if we just do cranial sacral therapy we are going to revert to our old ways of using the body, which is another reason why yoga, John Barnes' MFR and RFST can be of help.

Feldenkrais

This is a wonderful system to retrain the body in how to move. We typically use our bodies in a non-optimal way at least some of the time. We are often unaware of certain parts of our body, yet constantly aware of other parts of ourselves. We can overuse our bodies in a way that causes degeneration. Feldenkrais gives us an opportunity to reset how we use our body. It allows our unconscious to find easier, more optimal ways to move. We should be able to move without holding our breath or needing to breathe. We should be able to move our eyes without moving our head or our body, without jerkiness or holding our breath. Feldenkrais can make this easy.

Feldenkrais offers two modalities: the first is a group class called Awareness Through Movement (ATM) which helps us become aware of movement patterns. We can feel results in as little as an hour. The second form of treatment Feldenkrais practitioners offer is called Functional Integration (FI.) These are one-on-one sessions to help clients make changes in patterns of movement, thinking, sensing, and feeling. I've found them simple yet profound, non-invasive and energizing.

Some Feldenkrais practitioners are combining Functional Integration with energy work, which I have found helpful.

NuBax Trio and Gravity Boots

Reducing spinal tension is important. Our typical pattern with our primitive brain response to chronic stress causes back spasms and cramping as fascia and muscles contract. Chronic stress increases spinal tension. Excess tension in the fascia and muscles along our spine drives our vertebrae together in an unhealthy way. It's an unconscious reaction to emotional tension and to our primitive freeze response.

This excess fascial and muscle tension causes a reduced amount of blood flow in these critical areas. Bones, ligaments, tendons, muscle and fascia all suffer from poor circulation. I believe it's a contributing factor to osteoarthritis and osteoporosis, in part because not enough nutrients are being brought into the area, and cellular debris is not being efficiently cleared away.

I've used the Nubax Trio, a type of portable stretching device available online, to help get relief. The advantage of a Nubax is that the user doesn't have to hang upside down. Instead, the device is on the floor and one kneels over it to get the stretch.

Some people I know swear by regular use of gravity boots to help loosen up their backs.

If you are constantly in back pain, ask a chiropractor, osteopath or doctor to advise you on using one of these devices. The spine could be too degenerated to safely use one. If you get the okay, go slowly. The back can go into spasm if you try to do too much too soon. Once again, it's the build-up of fascia that causes the muscles to be painfully contracted, so while gravity boots or a Nubax Trio are of benefit, RFST and John Barne's MFR are also an important part of healing.

The Divided Mind

In the book *The Divided Mind* by Dr. John Sarno, he talks about what he has experienced in his work as a back doctor. Dr. Sarno has found that injured or degenerated spines are not painful once surgery has repaired the physical issue, if that's all that's going on. Most of the people he sees can be helped by treatment, but 10-15 percent cannot. Over the years, he's found that for these people, back pain is associated with the unconscious mind holding onto trauma and unprocessed anger. Highly sensitive people are continually stressed by their environments. They react more strongly to situations than others, and they take on other people's energy. They experience other people's emotional states as their own. As the years go by, they hold more and more and more tension in their bodies. They are much more stressed than the average person. He also found that highly sensitive people need a combination of psychotherapy and back treatment to end their back pain.

Sarno explains that this type of pain is a normal human response to feeling overwhelmed. Anyone can get to the same place by having enough trauma, even non-highly sensitive people. Studies have shown that only two days of interrupted REM sleep is enough to give people symptoms of fibromyalgia. I believe unconscious anger is worth addressing, because underneath that, I have found huge reservoirs of love. As we move through the emotions that are hard to face, like anger or fear, and take steps to activate the right brain, our acceptance of emotional states grows, leaving us more frequently in a state of non-judgment or peace.

If you are highly sensitive, remember it is not your fault. According to doctors, this is a genetic predisposition. People who are highly sensitive and who have experienced trauma either in childhood or as adults tend to have a lot of pain and health issues. There is a way back to health and happiness, and I'm here to tell you that I'm now consistently healthier and happier than I have ever been in my life.

Sleep Position

A word of caution about sleep position. Fascia grows day and night in response to thoughts, feelings and injuries. It is intended to strengthen us where we are weak. It's a common problem as we age that we are stiff when we wake up and I think the problem is connected to being mostly still in bed and fascia growing during sleep in response to dreams. It makes sense to me to be careful with our sleep position. I make sure my head is properly supported by a pillow. When I sleep on my side, my body weight is resting squarely on the side of my shoulder, not on the back edge. Alignment is important to keep one's shoulders from rolling forward. Bringing the legs up too much causes issues with digestion. I find I sleep better and have better digestion if my knees are no more than a ninety-degree angle to my body. I also notice that when my shins make a ninety-degree angle with my thighs or greater (so my feet are further away from my body) that I am much calmer and sleep better. Perhaps this is because when the knees and shins are drawn up and in too much, this mimics the classic shape of trauma—the fetal position. I used to have one knee drawn in higher than the other, which is also a stressful position that I don't recommend. It throws the body out of alignment and overactivates the psoas.

Action steps:
Easy:

Try a Feldenkrais class. The Seeing Clearly Workshop, which helps unlink breathing and vision from movement, is available online at feldenkraisinstitute.com, which also provides classes and therapists in New York City. You can also find an instructor near you at feldenkrais.com, as well as CDs for sale to walk you through training.

RFST also addresses pain, fascial tension and muscle imbalance, so I'd recommend *Resistance Flexibility 1.0.*

Moderate:

Make an appointment with a chiropractor, osteopathic physician or Feldenkrais practitioner for a one-on-one session and commit to regular self-care with them. If you are looking for what type of chiropractor might be best for you, I have found Gonstead to be very helpful for scoliosis for people in my family. Gonstead chiropractors work on specific regions of the spine that are stuck. They aim to bring back normal mobility to those regions. Sometimes chiropractic can bring too much mobility to areas that don't need it, and Gonstead avoids that issue. I'd recommend them for specific problems like scoliosis. The chiropractor that helped my family so much with scoliosis did not help my fibromyalgia. I know she is a gifted chiropractor, but none of her work decreased my pain, and she kept telling me that I should have been better long since. I began seeing other chiropractors who have helped me so much more. I think that for people who are not as in touch with their emotions, who are more thought-oriented, Gonstead is great, just like RFST is a great entry point for these thinking types. You can find a Gonstead chiropractor at gonstead.com. For people who are overly in touch with their emotions, or who have autoimmune issues, I'd suggest chiropractors who look to work with meridians and emotions. You'll need to interview your local chiropractors to see who is willing to work with you this way.

Harder:

Dr. John Sarno's findings are another reason to start counseling with a psychologist who is trained in Focusing or a Jungian analyst who uses dreams, active imagination, creative expression and Sandplay therapy in the tradition of Carl Jung and Dora Kalff to honor the body's wisdom. See contact details in Chapter 20's action steps.

Attend a group program offered by my friend Chad Cryder, author of *Men are DAWGS and Women are CATS: A Field Guide for Human Relationships*, and *A Great Love.* He's one of the coaches for the Angry Therapist's Catalyst Coaching Intensive Program. Chad is at chadcryder.com.

Chapter 10
Muscle-Based Therapies Relief

Trauma Release Process: Tremoring 101

David Berceli is a psychologist who travels the world giving people who've gone through unspeakable trauma the tools they need to heal. He's helped victims of the Bosnian War, the Rwandan Genocide, and the 2004 Indian Ocean tsunami disaster, among others. What he's learned to help them heal can help the rest of us heal.

He first stumbled across the problem when he was in Bosnia, where he noticed that babies were shaking in reaction to bomb blasts, but that the older children didn't shake as much. The older the children, the less they shook. The adults didn't show any reaction at all. It turns out they didn't want their children to know they were scared. In theory, this is admirable, but by not shaking, they were locking trauma in their bodies and teaching their children how to lock trauma in their own bodies. Older children were showing how "grownup" they were by hiding that response.

We also try to hide our stress or shock reaction in social situations and at work as a way of maintaining social status (and employment...) It's never too late to release trauma and it's something you can work on at home.

The Psoas

David Berceli's book talks about exercising just to the point of muscle fatigue and then allowing the muscles to tremor. He specifically talks about the psoas muscles and the muscles extending into the quadriceps and the inner thighs. Something he didn't mention that was very helpful to me was to put my hands against the headboard of my bed and press until my neck, shoulder and arm muscles fatigued and started to tremor. This released a lot of my fascial tension.

After completing the trauma release process, I had much less tension. I think it has contributed to my growing feeling of peace and calm. Occasionally I will have some tremoring after intense exercise, but it is nothing like the process in the initial years.

Muscles in spasm produce lactic acid, and I believe the combination with dense fascia traps much of the lactic acid in place. Anytime you have trigger points on your body or chronic pain in your back from muscle spasm, it's likely because there is a buildup of dense fascia, which makes the muscles too shortened. The fascia is locking the muscles in place and is doing most of the muscles' work. Once the fascia is released, I've found the muscle is quite weak. At that point, I need to rebuild my muscle strength. I now expect it as part of the process. I get excited when I experience this, because I know I'm making progress in healing. Fascia release happens at different levels. Fascia is constantly being formed, so it's a work-in-process to head towards reduced fascial tension, not a one-shot deal.

Getting Muscles Functioning Correctly

When fascia is released it allows the muscle to move, proper blood flow gets going and lactic acid gets released. When I first started hot yoga, I would hit a point in a class where I would feel nauseated. I realized it was an overload of lactic acid, which is processed by the liver, and I needed to back off how much stretch I was doing so that my liver could adjust.

While working on the trauma release process I got to the point where the tremors weren't noticeable if others were to look at me. Once that happened, I started adding it into my hot yoga practice. I'd spend an extra few minutes at the end of the session as we were lying flat on our backs in Savasana to let the tremors subside.

If you try releasing muscle-based tension and find tremoring makes you too uncomfortable or anxious, get assistance before continuing. At times, this and all the other release therapies have made me feel uncomfortable or overwhelmed. Seeing a psychologist was a great help to me as I went through the healing process.

Qigong and TaiChi

Qigong is a wonderful system of body movement. I had a teacher who helped me clear my entire system, bringing in fresh energy and finding out which meridian pathways were currently blocked. What a wonderful gift. Qigong masters can get us into quite an in-depth connection to our body during a class. In Santa Barbara, I've been lucky to take classes with Master Li Jungfen, who teaches worldwide through shengzhen.org.

Tai Chi is also wonderful for moving chi (another term for energy) in the body. Like Qigong, it is also helpful with moving lymph through the body and helping us connect to our body.

Before I started these alternative methods of healing, I used to get at least two or three migraines a month. Vision therapy helped to reduce both the frequency and severity of my migraines. The process of meditation and taking classes in Qigong and Tai Chi helped me understand how much holding I was still doing. In addition, learning Touch for Health and PanHarmonic Healing, which I'll go in depth on in Chapter 15, has given me tools to release energy rather than hold it in my body. Being able to move energy through these different methods so I do not hold it and develop a migraine has been invaluable.

Resistance Flexibility Strength Training

As mentioned before, I have found RFST to be an effective form of stretching with resistance. I mention it here because the workout it provides allows tremoring too. Again, the meridian pathways reach through a lot of different muscles. Blockage along these channels can cause pain in the muscles they are paired with, which leads to an inflammatory pathway. Working with self-stretches, assisted and/or trainer stretching, I get an increased sensation of energy flow, lightness and ease of being. Activating muscles while stretching allows fascia to release and muscles to elongate.

Massage

Massage has also been a big help for me. The benefits from it are that trigger points can be calmed and the muscles that are in constant overuse for weeks, months or years get a chance to get rid of some of the lactic acid buildup. Massage that focuses on fascia can help allow the muscles to release rather than being chronically contracted. Chronic contraction is both inflammatory and painful. Massage also improves circulation.

I enjoy massages that are meridian-based, though others can find it overwhelming. I like Thai massage because it combines massage with meridian-based stretching. I found that during Thai massage I tended to have a lot of tremoring, which releases tension, stretches fascia and brings about healthier blood flow. I also find meridian-based Chinese massage very helpful.

Rolfing was an amazing process of releasing fascia and allowing me to utilize my body better. Dense fascia had bound my shoulder blades to my back ribs and locked my hips out of alignment. My right collarbone didn't move properly, so my lungs couldn't expand fully. Despite what I'd heard about the discomfort of Rolfing, my Rolfer, Torrey Trover, was intent on keeping me comfortable. My first Rolfing session was an overview which included some visceral massage, which releases fascia from around the internal organs. That day, I learned firsthand from Rolfing how emotions get locked in the body, frozen in time. As the fascia was released, I re-experienced the emotion from a basketball being slammed in my stomach when I was eight. By paying attention to the feelings of both body sensation and emotional responses, I could process and release that trauma.

Chi Nei Tsang & Transformational Abdominal Massage

Chi Nei Tsang is a type of Chinese massage that is an applied form of Qigong. Chi Nei Tsang believes that, in essence, emotions are organs and organs are emotions. This type of massage helps to clear the abdomen of unprocessed emotional charges. My masseuse, Jada Delaney, has developed a process beyond Chi Nei Tsang that she calls Transformational Abdominal Massage (TAM.) TAM helps people change how they manage life from the inside, so they can experience more energy, better physical health and greater joy. I have found it to be wonderfully therapeutic.

Action steps:

Easy:

If you have not been severely traumatized, read David Berceli's book, *The Revolutionary Trauma Release Process: Transcend Your Toughest Times* and begin to work through the exercises. (If you have been severely traumatized, please read the Harder section below.)

Moderate:

Find a masseuse to help support your work in calming your trigger points or accumulated held stress.

Try a Rolfing massage—and if you find someone who works well with you, try "the Ten", a series of ten massages designed to maximize releasing fascia-holding throughout your body in a balanced way. See Torrey if you're in Santa Barbara. She can be reached at torrey.trover@gmail.com.

Try working with a visceral masseuse or someone who does Chi Nei Tsang massage. See Jada in Santa Barbara or San Francisco for TAM, she can be reached at jadadelaney.cmt@gmail.com.

Harder:

If you have been severely traumatized, find a good psychologist who can help you heal, then with your psychologist's blessing, begin to work through Berceli's book, or find someone who does Somatic Experiencing (SE) as developed by Peter Levine, author of *Waking the Tiger*. SE comes highly recommended, but I have yet to try it myself because I found the healing I needed earlier in my journey. In researching it for the book, I came across Irene Lyon, who has a program to help heal the nervous system that combines Feldenkrais with SE, among other things. The program has an active community and offers 3 free videos that are right on point. If this sounds interesting, check out the videos and see if it sounds like it's your path. She can be reached at irenelyon.com.

Try classes in Qigong, Tai Chi or Jin Shin Do to see what works best for you.

If any of the processes in this chapter seem emotionally overwhelming when you try them, find a psychologist who specializes in Focusing or one who does Jungian analysis incorporating dreams, active imagination, creative expression and Sandplay. Contact details for Sandplay and Jungian analysts are in the Action steps of Chapter 20.

Chapter 11
More Myofascial Help

John Barnes Myofascial Release Method

John Barnes is a physical therapist who is a leading expert in myofascial release (MFR.) He has centers in Sedona, Arizona and Malvern, Pennsylvania. Because he's trained over 100,000 healthcare professionals (mostly PTs and masseuses) in his methods, it should not be hard to find someone in your area who is experienced in this method to help you.

The core idea of his method is that fascia is moldable and can change shape. That sounded like a good way to work on my fascial tension, so I booked an appointment in Ventura, California with a local expert in this method, a masseuse named Cindy Rowland Wilson. The first treatment was soothing and calming. As she walked me through the treatment, she encouraged me to feel into my body as she held my ankles. She asked me to feel where it was tight and imagine that it was softening or melting. I visualized melting candle wax and warm taffy being pulled and after a few minutes, I could feel the region softening and becoming more mobile. She then continued to my arms, gently moving them and letting them release, again asking me for internal visualization help. It occurred to me to begin Focusing (see Chapter 20 for details) as part of the process, which I found to be a great pairing. Cindy explained that she only did a gentle release, to give me a taste of the method. She encouraged me to do a specific type of stretching at home and suggested some books for further explanation. She said a full treatment often makes those with fibromyalgia feel like they've taken two steps forward and one step back. She suggested thinking of it as a process of healing, not a cure-in-a-day. After trying the technique at home and seeing great results, I've added it to my daily routine.

Releasing Fascial Constrictions for Improved Lymphatic Flow

Among other things that Cindy has taught me, MFR addresses fascial constrictions in the breasts. I never thought I'd use that technique, but it's been helpful because at times I feel breast constriction when I sleep on my stomach. Using the release technique alleviates the discomfort. Because it feels less restricted, I think that the breast tissue is likely getting better blood and lymph flow. This seems like a good thing to me, so I thought I'd suggest it as a tool to ask your MFR therapist for, should you feel constrictions.

The Orbi Therapy Ball

Another useful tip that Cindy gave me was the importance of using an Orbi therapy ball to help release fascia (you can find it online at theorbi.com), or make one by putting two racquetballs into a tube sock, tying it tightly and cutting off any excess material once you're satisfied with it. I don't think there's anything I've tried that's been more important than working with the Orbi daily. I would not have known how to correctly use one without first going to a John Barnes' MFR specialist for at least a few sessions. If I wake up in the night, I reach for the Orbi and start working on the points that have the most tension. It helps me to fall back to sleep more quickly, and over time it's helped significantly reduce my high fascial tension.

Keep in mind that muscles that are relaxed should feel soft. If you touch a relaxed muscle and it feels gristly, hard or tender, it's likely to have dense fascia in it.

In the months since I began this treatment, I've also seen Lisa West in Ventura, a PT who filled in when Cindy was away. Lisa is another skilled healer who's working on a book based on her experience as a therapist and I've counted myself lucky to be in her care, too.

The Difference between MFR and RFST

John Barnes' MFR is perfect for people who are not inclined to exertion. RFST requires an effort at physicality and it's easier for people who are in shape. That said, RFST breaks up excess fascia and John Barnes' MFR has us live with our excess fascia. John Barnes' MFR helps us reshape it so it no longer binds, but it remains (free of restrictions.) I think there's a place for both types of treatments, and I'm glad to have access to both.

My first workshop in MFR was with Lori Zeltwanger, a long-time MFR practitioner who travels nationwide with her training programs. She offers a 5-day immersion retreat twice a year, one in California, the other in Florida. It was a wonderful experience for both newbies like myself as well as the therapists who attended.

Cindy recommended an excellent book called *Comprehensive Myofascial Self Treatment*, by Joyce Karnis. In the book, Karnis discusses the dura, the deepest layer of the fascial system. The dural tube is a thick sheath that surrounds the brain and spinal cord all the way down to the tailbone. Karnis says common conditions that can be improved with treatment of the dural system include headaches, neck pain, back and tailbone pain, brain fog, decreased concentration and memory, depression, anxiety, muscle tone, tremors, numbness and tingling. That piqued my interest, because it's a laundry list of fibromyalgia symptoms.

Dural Tube Stretching

Eventually, my skill level at receiving treatment was good enough that when Cindy did a dural tube (also called a dural sheath) stretch, I could let go. She did the neck release on page 68 of Karnis's book, holding my head up for me. Over the next few weeks, I followed up with extended plow position poses in my hot yoga class and I've felt the sheath releasing more and more. It is helping to reset how jammed my upper cervical bones are into my brainstem. My chiropractor has joked that my C1 vertebra was so tight that it was on its way to my ears. I think whiplash or multiple falls leads to dural sheath tightness, which leads to fibromyalgia—and that the dural sheath being so tight disturbs sleep and puts too much stress on the neck vertebrae, jamming them into the brain stem. C1, also known as the Atlas, is connected to nerves that control the blood supply to the head, pituitary gland, scalp, bones of the face, brain, inner ear, middle ear and sympathetic nervous system. Possible symptoms of a misalignment of C1 include headaches, nervousness, insomnia, head colds, high blood pressure, migraines, nervous breakdowns, amnesia, chronic tiredness and dizziness. The dural sheath can also be impacted by whiplash and falls on the tailbone. There are exercises to release that too. I'd like to suggest that along with developing the mind/body connection as outlined in this book, that once the initial spinal injury is healed, patients be encouraged to start doing dural sheath release exercises with an MFR specialist to help avoid developing fibromyalgia. Check with your chiropractor or doctor, MFR specialist or physical therapist first.

Holistic Pulsing (I know, what a name! but it works)

I first came across Holistic Pulsing (HP) at the weeklong Focusing Summer Institute I attended in 2016 where a teacher named Marieke Hoeve from Holland taught it to our group. HP is more commonly known in Europe and New Zealand, and is done by practitioners who specialize in it.

During treatment, practitioners use gentle rocking to see where the body does not move freely. They spend time in those congested areas to help free tension and balance the body.

Holistic Pulsing feels like the gentle rocking I did as a child when I tried to soothe myself to sleep. It's an easy skill to learn and a great one to have in your toolkit. It immediately helped me sleep more soundly. We learned how to work with different areas of the body each day, but the highlight came at the end of the week, when Marieke taught us to combine it with Focusing (see Chapter 20.)

I mentioned Focusing in an earlier chapter and it combines well with multiple modalities. Combining it with Holistic Pulsing immediately led to tremoring release in my pelvic floor muscles. Many of us hold excess tension in our pelvic floor without ever being aware of it. (More details about the pelvic floor below.)

The Pelvic Floor—If You Have a Pelvic Floor, You Need to Read This (trust me, you have one.)

The pelvic floor is a set of muscles at the base of the abdomen, attached to the pelvis. These muscles need to be strong to have proper bladder and bowel control among other things.

Overall, one in four women will have pelvic floor problems during their lifetime. The risk increases with age. By age 80, almost half of all women will have experienced a pelvic floor disorder. Men have a lower risk, but can also have pelvic floor problems.

I struggled with pelvic floor tension for more than five years before getting correctly diagnosed. Many factors can cause pelvic floor problems. For me, it was a combination of falling off a wall at age seven, a bike at age seventeen, the whiplash car accident at thirty-nine and then becoming a spin biking enthusiast in my forties. Instructors often don't correct for poor form, nor do they do proper stretching to release the pelvic floor after a class. It's common for women who have had Cesarean sections to have a problem because weakened abdominal muscles make it very difficult to hold the correct form through the course of a spin bike workout. Over time, this leads to excessive use of pelvic floor muscles and tightening of both muscles and fascia. Women who deliver vaginally have increased risk for pelvic floor problems, too. Men are likely to develop problems from heavy lifting, or from having pelvic surgery for prostate cancer.

Pelvic Floor Dysfunction
Pelvic floor dysfunction can be missed because it mimics so many other problems. My gynecologist was sure I needed estrogen cream,

when I really needed pelvic floor therapy. I couldn't identify the pain I was having, only that it was a stinging and burning kind of pain that turned out to be caused by muscle spasms. Stress in my life made the muscle spasms worse. Even more confusing for me, I would go to the pelvic floor therapist for treatment, then encounter a stressful experience at home and in less than five minutes I'd feel the stress undo the benefits of the treatment.

Accidents and Falls Add Up

For either gender, being in an accident that unseats the spine from its pelvic base can contribute to the problem, whether it's multiple falls, like people with cerebral palsy often suffer from, or a fall from a bike or a car accident. My physical therapist, Dr. Betty Gao of Westchester Physical Therapy, explained that the pelvis has several notches in it to keep the spine seated in the event of a heavy fall. The spine can slip and reseat itself, but once the spine is even minimally off center, the muscles on the opposite side at the base must contract to keep the vertebra vertical. The next vertebra will be impacted in the other direction as opposing muscles try to keep it from continuing too far in the direction of the vertebra below it, and so on and on.

According to Dr. Gao, these muscles are constantly in spasm, releasing lactic acid and prostaglandins among other chemicals. Once the prostaglandin levels become high enough, it goes systemic (circulating throughout the body) and the body starts to attack itself. That's one way autoimmune illness begins.

What I've learned from RFST and from MFR, as well as Focusing, is that the fascia we create from our thoughts and feelings about sex, about any sexual trauma, or about past sexual partners can stay with us until we do the MFR or RFST work to release it. In particular, the fascia around the psoas, our fight-or-flight response muscle that pulls us into a fetal position, connects to the pelvic floor fascia, so I believe it could potentially impact the ability to achieve erection in men (perhaps by interfering with blood flow) or orgasm in women (which requires the ability of muscles to release and work in tandem.)

Women, Fascia and Orgasm

Women need to have low enough fascial tension so that their muscles can tense further in order to have an orgasm. If resting fascial tone is too high, women have difficulty having an orgasm. There are a lot of conflicting messages for women around sex in our society, which can generate a lot of inner conflict and tension.

Fascia and scar tissue builds up because of accidents, thoughts, feelings, and trauma. It's possible to treat the health issues that come up through a variety of ways, which I've listed below under the action steps at the end of this chapter.

If this is an issue, please remember that this is a process. The first step is becoming aware, and that's huge. I hope you feel encouraged now that you know more about where to focus your energies in order to heal.

Action steps:
Easy:

Try Holistic Pulsing to reduce pelvic floor tension.

Google YouTube videos for demonstrations of Holistic Pulsing.

Read *Gentle Miracles: Holistic Pulsing* by Tovi Browning.

Femfusionfitness has an easy half hour video of pelvic floor stretches: http://femfusionfitness.com/pelvic-release-stretches/

Moderate:

Try RFST and John Barnes' MFR to reduce fascia and fascial tension.

Read Bob Cooley's *Resistance Flexibility 1.0* and John Barnes' *Healing Ancient Wounds*.

Find a pelvic floor therapist who uses MFR.

Take steps to reduce the stress levels in your life. Meditation and yoga are good choices, as is marriage counseling or changing jobs.

Harder:

Consider John Barnes' centers in Arizona or Pennsylvania. More at myofascialrelease.com

Try a workshop with Lori Zeltwanger. You can find out more info at her website advancedreleasetherapy.com.

Look into Holistic Pulsing training and attend a training program. Most of what I've found is available through Holland, the UK and New Zealand. You can reach Marieke Hoeve at mariekehoeve@upcmail.nl.

Find an RFST trainer to work with at geniusofflexibility.com.

Dr. Betty Gao has a private physical therapy practice in Sleepy Hollow, NY. Her office can be reached at 914-909-6970.

Wednesday:

Stop Reliving Emotions

Chapter 12
Emotions Made Easy

What Emotions Are For

Our emotions are a survival mechanism to help process often bewildering environmental and social cues to maximize our chance of survival—both physically and socially. The emotional brain is an add-on to the primitive reptilian brain, but the two brains don't always work well together.

Primitive Brain Response

Having an emotional brain is an evolutionary advantage, but there is a problem with it: the primitive brain cannot tell the difference between an actual event and an imagined one. All those times we imagined being a hero, or got angry and stewed about the way we were treated at school or work, reinventing our response over and over again in our minds, our primitive brain was pumping out adrenaline as if it were real. When we relive a traumatic or shaming event that happened to us, our primitive brain pumps out the adrenaline needed as if it were happening all over again.

That adrenaline is made in a factory (our body) that has limited resources. When we overproduce adrenaline, we have fewer resources to produce other necessary neurotransmitters. In addition, producing too much adrenaline creates an inflammatory process and chronic inflammation leads to disease. So how do we cope with emotions?

Ninety Second Rule

According to neurologist/researcher Dr. Jill Bolte Taylor, emotions are a chemical response process that only last ninety seconds. Any further emotional reaction comes from a person choosing to stay in that emotional loop. In other words, emotions "only" last for ninety seconds—if you understand how to step out of the emotional loop, by accepting them so they can be processed, learned from, and released. Those ninety seconds can ramp up into something so excruciating that some people will resort to anything: drugs, alcohol, you name it, to avoid it because those emotions keep coming back. It's not a conscious decision. Our unconscious primitive brain is terrified. It's a pattern that starts in childhood and continues into adulthood. Avoiding emotion stores it and begins an inflammatory pathway. I've read that the actual biochemical process of getting rid of the emotional chemicals from our system can take up to 20 minutes. In my life, I was so scared of emotions like fear, anger and sadness that I avoided them all, rationalized them away, and got sick.

Lots of people use sports or hobbies in healthy ways to process emotions. They tune into the flow they feel from engaging in them and release stress that way. Sports like surfing, playing golf or tennis come to mind, as do hobbies like gardening, collecting model trains, and knitting. A Cardiff University survey found that 81% of respondents with depression claimed that knitting made them happier. These are all wonderful ways to process emotion. They're also an opportunity to add tension to ourselves by being competitive about it or forcing a fit with an activity (perhaps because of family or peer pressure) when it's not really our cup of tea. Be sure to choose something that brings you joy.

My Best Pathways to Process Emotion

There are lots of pathways I've found to make me braver so I can cope with emotion. The first one is meditation. I am not talking about the kind of meditation where I gaze at my navel and start chanting. There are completely left-brain ways to do meditation. I've combined the best practices I've learned into a meditation practice which processes emotions out of the body. Once I had the tools to release my emotions, it was a heck of a lot easier to confront them and allow my chronic stress to begin to release.

Separating From my Thoughts and Feelings

Meditation made me realize that there is a part of me that was not caught up in my emotional experience and I could call on it to help me choose another path. The part of me that was not caught up in my emotional experience was my right brain. I can access it during times of trauma or stress. The right brain is always peaceful. Listening to Dr. Jill Bolte Taylor's TED Talk, "My Stroke of Insight" and reading her book helped me understand better about the right brain.

It can be cathartic to vent emotions, but my emotional self is not always the kindest or smartest part of myself. I would do better to call on that other peaceful part of myself to calmly take over in times of stress.

Meditation helps to strengthen the awareness and connection to that other self which resides in the prefrontal cortex. When our reptilian brain or emotional brain sends threat messages, we have a small window of time to choose our response. Once we respond with these more primitive areas, we get caught up in the emotion of the situation and can no longer easily access our prefrontal cortex. Our default survival mechanism makes us shift into using our more ancient brain systems.

By meditating, I'm allowing my brain to become better able to discern between a true emergency and situations where it's safe to stay in my prefrontal cortex. Ultimately our highest and best human selves lay in the prefrontal cortex, fully in touch with our compassionate emotions while acknowledging our own needs.

We want to spend more time in that kind of head space. Meditation reduces inflammation, because it stimulates the parasympathetic nervous system when we are in this state. A world full of people doing their best to achieve mastery in the practice of meditation would truly be a beautiful place.

Primary Storage is in Our Brain, Secondary Storage is in our Body

The second pathway I found to help make me braver in dealing with emotions was to realize that I needed to feel the emotions in my body for them to be processed and released, and that there was a way I could do this that hurt less than just waiting for emotions to hit me unprepared. I had a big backlog of unprocessed emotions, but I figured that if I took on clearing a little of my suppressed emotions every day I'd be reducing that inflammatory neurochemical stockpile. That meant literally noticing where emotions started and where they moved to within my body. I noticed muscle twitches and energy movement as well as feelings.

Seven Ways to Help Process Emotions

There are seven effective ways I've found to help process emotions. The first is with specialized kinesiology (see chapter 15), the second is with Focusing (see chapter 20), the third is MFR, the fourth is RFST, the fifth is yoga, the sixth is holistic pulsing, and the seventh is dance. I was completely closed to trying anything to do with specialized kinesiology for the first forty-nine years of my life. I only became open to it because of being sick enough, and that was only after trying everything else first. The other six things are much more mainstream, so if you have a similar mindset against trying alternative health remedies, try the others first.

When I was at my sickest, I realized I had become so avoidant of emotions that I rarely felt any. Instead, I felt varying amounts of pain, numbness and tingling when I got upset; it depended on my stress levels just how bad the symptoms were. It took a lot of effort to learn to tune into my body for the fleeting sensations I was still capable of. Our emotional brain sends out neuropeptides into our body and they lodge in specific regions. We even have expressions for this: "He's got a lot of gall." "She vented her spleen." "I didn't have the stomach for it." Folk wisdom understood there was a connection between these organs and certain emotions.

Emotions are Part of a Cycle

There is another downside to avoiding emotions. Eventually blocking the negative ones meant I blocked the positive ones too, because they are part of a cycle. This was first realized by traditional Chinese medicine. In my case, because I rejected anger, I couldn't feel joy. I had reduced the energy available to run on the fire element—those nerves that run through the heart, small intestine, pericardium, thyroid, adrenals and their related muscles. This in turn interrupted flow through the rest of the meridian system.

We each have our emotional signature, depending on which emotions we were allowed to express when we were growing up. Within each family we were assigned a role which often had to do with our birth order. That emotional signature is a mix of blocked meridian pathways, where we've resisted the neuropeptides' messages, and opened meridian pathways, where we've allowed their messages.

Calming Our Emotional Mind

I think we need to learn both how to calm our emotional mind and to fully feel our held emotions in order to reach optimal health. If we ignore or avoid feeling our emotions, they persist. Because of how scared our primitive brain can get, many people act as if bad emotions are "it" in a game of hide and go seek, as if all we have to do is run away to win the game.

When scary, strong emotions show up, I think of it as getting blasted by hot or cold water in an unexpected shower. We can figure out how to adjust the shower head and try to find a safe corner to stand in, but eventually a crisis hits that means the water blasts stronger than we've ever experienced. There's nowhere to go in the shower that isn't getting hit. In times of crisis, the drain gets stuck shut. During hard times, the tub seems to get deeper and deeper until we are swimming in it. It gets exhausting when lots of bad stuff happens at once and all we're doing is treading water without rest.

At times like these we feel like we are drowning in emotions. We can get so exhausted, so tired, and be in so much pain that we just want it to end. That is when some people think about committing suicide, when they've lost hope and just cannot take all the fear, anger, shame, and loss. Life feels too exhausting to continue.

There are solutions. There always have been, we just need find them and learn how to let those emotions drain off—-which is what I call processing. Committing to positive self-talk is important. When my boys were very young, every morning I would take them downstairs and hold them up to the windows of the front door. As they looked out, I would say, "It's a brand-new day. Every day is a brand-new day, filled with hope and new possibilities." As much as I was mothering them in a positive way, I was parenting myself too, focusing on the positives in my life, rather than the exhaustion from lack of sleep to care for them in the night, the worries about my health, the unraveling of my marriage. What kind of positive self-talk can you add to your life?

Emotions Contain Information that Increase Odds of our Survival

Nothing is wasted by the emotional brain. Since emotional neuropeptides carry information that helps increase our odds of survival and are stored in our bodies for processing later, I think of us as having primary memory storage in our brain and a backup system for storage in our body.

There are situations when it is not possible to feel and express our emotions fully in real time, like in school or at work. But it's important to process emotions later, no matter how much time has passed. It gives us a chance to reset and calm down, so we're not so triggered the next time we go to school or work.

Unless They are Processed Negative Emotions Add up Over Time

Whether we have come to toxic emotional storage through major trauma or through the thousands of slights of daily life, they add up in the same way when they are ignored or avoided. Unprocessed neurochemicals are lodged in our body until our bodies are overflowing with them. Either way will cause the same pathway of disease to begin, it's just a matter of how early in our life they'll show up.

For me, the easiest and most complete emotional reset happens through specialized kinesiology (more details in Chapter 15) because I can do it anywhere—in bed, or in the car. The second easiest is meditation because again, I can do parts of it anywhere, anytime. The third easiest is MFR because I can do that in bed too if I wake up. The fourth is RFST because I have to get out of bed to avoid disturbing my partner. You'll have your own unique preferences.

Questioning our thoughts

I was raised believing that others' actions were responsible for how I felt. I didn't understand that my life experiences created a pattern for how I would react to other people's actions. That meant I had responsibility for how I reacted. As Jack Canfield says in *The Success Principles*, 'you must take 100% responsibility for your life, no excuses, blaming or complaining.' Someone once said, 'holding onto resentment is like drinking poison and expecting the other person to die.' I could learn to forgive because I could see how another person with a different history might have a different reaction. It's important to forgive for our own benefit—since resentment is an inflammatory emotion. If someone is mistreating us, it's also important that we take steps to protect ourselves, since abuse will also cause an inflammatory response. Best is if we forgive and get out of situations like that.

Sometimes others mistreat us because they get energy from the ill-will they provoke in others. Perhaps it's because they learned that negative attention is better than no attention at all. Regardless of why, it's damaging to ourselves to respond in kind, especially if we are sick. I've found it's best to disengage and think neutral thoughts until I can move on with my day.

I was also raised to need everyone's approval and if I didn't get it, I was crushed. I didn't understand that even the nicest people have people who are critical of them. As Canfield states in *The Success Principles*, 'it's none of our business what other people think of us.' If we make it our business, it becomes toxic to our health. I've learned the hard way to act out of love and if other people misunderstand me and won't change their opinion of me, at least I've tried my best.

Questioning my thoughts and feelings has been an important tool for me to stop being a victim and start being an advocate for myself. It also helps reduce the repetitive thinking and resultant emotional whirlwind I experience, which lowers the stress and inflammation in the primitive and emotional parts of my brain. As I mentioned in Chapter 8, another tool for emotions that won't release is to hand them off in prayer. You don't have to believe in God; just try it and you might find that you can benefit from it too. Chalk it up to the powers of the human brain if you're an atheist.

Action steps:
Easy:
Find a meditation program you like; see my suggestions from Chapter 5.

Read *The Success Principles* and choose a few items at a time to work on.

Moderate:
Take a meditation class that combines writing to heal exercises with Bön breathwork to tire the body and process and release the energy of emotions. I offer that combination in my programs; others may too.

Find an MFR practitioner near you at myofascialrelease.com and get a treatment.

Take an RFST class, buy the book or try out the videos available at thegeniusofflexibility.com.

Buy a Touch for Health Manual (the original version of specialized kinesiology for home use) and read it.

Find a yoga program you enjoy and go to extra classes when you're particularly stressed.

Try a dance class that makes you feel happy and attend classes regularly.

Harder:

Take a class in Touch for Health, Brain Gym ®, or PanHarmonic Healing (other forms of specialized kinesiology), where you'll learn how to do muscle testing and give energy balances for yourself, family and friends. See Chapter 15 action steps for contact details.

Chapter 13
Beyond Processing Emotions

Finding Bliss in Negative Emotions

There's a little secret I discovered after learning meditation, mindfulness, specialized kinesiology (see chapter 15) and Focusing (see chapter 20.) Often when I connect to my feelings every morning and welcome them even if they're negative, after about 5-10 minutes of being with it, I find myself in bliss. It doesn't matter how crappy the feelings are. I can start off fearful, angry, depressed and end up in joy. It took me a while to realize that only once emotions are truly welcomed, can they be fully felt and processed. Once that happens, our mind and body are at peace with each other and peace equals bliss. That's the right-brain non-judgmental state I'm connecting to. For many years I was hiding from the ability to feel bliss. How sad is that? At least I've learned the secret now. There's a caveat to this: if our feelings are painful, we can dissociate when we are first learning to connect with our emotions. It's an unconscious process, meaning we don't know we are doing it; our unconscious takes over to protect us. Dissociating, which means detaching from and trying to avoid the emotional experience we are having, can also make us feel calmer and sleepy. Dissociating is a common coping mechanism. I think of a little dissociating as being a tool because there is only so much emotional and mental pain human beings can handle at a time. How useful is it to know that when your mind/body have had enough, they will deflect you from the pain? Because then with your toolkit you can choose to work on the pain a little at a time until you are comfortable trusting that it won't get overwhelming.

Meditation, Mindfulness and Specialized Kinesiology's use of Acupressure

I am grateful for meditation and mindfulness because they gave me tools to separate from my emotional state and learn that there was a part of me that was always okay and could be reset to calm, even when I was suffering from an emotional storm. Ultimately meditation and mindfulness are only a part of the toolkit. If I have an urgent emotional message from my body I can move into Focusing to get to an understanding of what my body is trying to express. Or else I can use acupressure points from specialized kinesiology (Chapter 15) to process it. I've found that I don't consciously need to know everything that the body and unconscious are processing—the big stuff always makes itself known. The rest of it is processed and learned from by my body/mind so I can have access to it later if it needs to become conscious.

Questioning Your Thoughts

Tools like these are handy in life, so that we can catch ourselves when we separate from being happy and joyful. One of the downfalls of our culture is the tendency to think we'll be happy when some goal is met, like once we finish college or get a high-paying job, buy a house or have children, or retire. It's been clear from research done on this that achieving goals has little lasting impact on our happiness. That's because when we achieve our goals, we develop a new normal and our grasping mental state wants more. As Marci Shimoff says in her book *Happy for No Reason*, "question your thoughts, because your thoughts aren't always true. Judging, worrying, overthinking, dwelling on the bad, and focusing on the negative stimulates areas of the brain involved in depression and anxiety. If instead, we think positively, accept and trust the good in our lives and savor it, it's calming to our brain." After reading her book, I made it a point to change my mindset. I focus on happiness now. Gratitude is what I turn to whenever I start down a negative path. I remember to forgive rather than continue with an overthinking spree. It's not an easy change because, as I've said before, human beings are judgment machines. Our brains are hardwired for judgment when we're stressed. Even when not stressed, many of us habitually revert to unconscious patterns handed down from our parents and their parents rather than thinking for ourselves. Having the tools to cope with the emotions that come up when we question our default response is vital for clear thinking. So is remembering our intention of heading towards positivity. The more chronically stressed we are, the more ill we are, the more important it is to make the change.

Progress, not Perfection

I'm human, so all I'm capable of is progress, not perfection. Even so, these attempts at progress that I make daily have helped change my life. Here's an example from my life; perhaps you can think of something recent in your life that you could try this type of response on:

I had an appointment for a Thursday afternoon with a specialist in Los Angeles to see if I needed a root canal. I live a two-hour drive away. The charger prongs on my cell phone were broken, so I bought a wireless charger for the drive down until I could get my phone replaced. I got to LA with 30% battery power from using the phone to navigate; something was wrong with the wireless charger, too. I charged the phone the entire time I was in LA, but didn't realize the Near Field Communications setting was off, preventing it from charging properly. I had an emergency root canal and left the office in the dark during rush hour in LA with 13% battery power. I think a lot of women might relate to feeling vulnerable in a situation like that. The GPS led me in a direction I didn't recognize. I caught myself thinking thoughts like, "this is the worst!" "oh my gosh, this is so dangerous!" before catching myself and remembering that times like that are where I'm supposed to be finding my happiness. My first cynical thought was, "yeah right, but this is an impossible situation!" I knew I had to turn my thinking around. I reminded myself that since I didn't know the outcome, I couldn't know how dangerous it truly was. It was dangerous only if I got stranded without GPS, and only then if I got unlucky about where I got stranded. Most people are helpful and kind. Until the worst happens, it might be dangerous, but it might not be. I know it's better for my brain and my health if I can keep myself from going to the worst possible scenario, so I turned off survival mode by starting to be grateful for what I had: I was warm, had a reliable car and a full tank of gas. Once I started thinking that way, rational thoughts started showing up. I realized how lucky I was, because I only needed the power to last until I got to the 405 freeway—I could find my own way home from there. It also occurred to me that if I ran out of power, the charger seemed to work if I kept moving the phone around to restart it, so I could park and idle the car if necessary until I had enough charge. Thinking those thoughts quickly got me out of high-alert mode and into adventure mode. Not long afterwards, I realized I'd shifted into feeling happy. I made it to the 405 just fine. Being aware of the dangers and treating them as reality can create epigenetic changes to our cells that make us live in chronic stress. Being mindful that there are choices in how I think and that I can redirect myself to healthier brain chemistry has been the key to going beyond merely reacting to my thoughts and emotions. If you're interested, think of ways this could work in your life.

Action steps:
Easy:
    Find meditation and mindfulness programs you like; see my suggestions from Chapter 5.

Moderate:
    Read Eugene Gendlin's book *Focusing*. Read Bebe Simon's *How I Teach Focusing: Discovering the Gift of Your Inner Wisdom*. Attend a training program in Focusing. Find a Focusing partner through

focusing.org.

Harder:

Take a course in Touch for Health, Brain Gym ®, or PanHarmonic Healing (contact details in action steps of Chapter 15), where you'll learn how to do muscle testing and give energy balances for yourself, family and friends.

Find a therapist who uses Focusing to help give you insight into your inner guidance at focusing.org

Chapter 14
Acupuncture

The Benefits of Acupuncture

Over the course of my life, I've gone from thinking I'd never even want to try acupuncture to being very grateful for its existence. I first used it to help me get pregnant—as a support for donor egg in vitro—and successfully carry my twins to term.

There's been a lot of research showing the benefits of acupuncture. It's been clinically shown to reduce pain, improve sleep and digestion, as well as one's general sense of well-being. It's also been shown to help nausea, migraine headache, anxiety, depression, insomnia, and infertility. It's been proven to help allergic rhinitis and hay fever, dysentery, menstrual cramps, facial pain and TMJ, hypertension, hypotension, knee pain, low back pain, morning sickness, vomiting, rheumatoid arthritis, sciatica, postoperative pain, stroke, and sprains.

I've also used acupuncture to help improve digestion and immune function. I feel it's been an important part of my healing.

I learned about Five Elements Acupuncture in the past year. It uses specific points to help release where we hold emotion in the body. These points are called Windows to the Sky. Practitioners who treat using this method give sessions which support work being done with a psychologist.

My practitioner asks what is going on in my life and how I've been, both regarding health and pain, but also emotionally. I tell him the condensed version of what is going on in my psychologist sessions, dreams and kinesiology sessions and he bases his treatment on that. I've found it very helpful to use this type of acupuncture. The other type of treatment which he does that helps with pain is cupping—heating the air inside specially designed bottles and running them along my back. I end up with some bruising at times, but it helps locked fascia to release, which also helps make me feel more mobile.

I've also gotten a lot of help from Pamela Grant, an acupuncturist who is also a Shengzen Qigong teacher in Santa Barbara. She does a lymphatic drainage treatment that works wonders.

Action steps:

Easy: find a good local acupuncturist.

Moderate: find a 5 Elements practitioner if needed.

Harder: If you're ever in Santa Barbara, CCOM is run by Mark Sherwood and Nicki Doner Sherwood. You can reach them at yourccom.com. Pamela Grant is at pamela-grant.com.

Chapter 15
Specialized Kinesiology

The Benefits of Specialized Kinesiology

The same type of acupressure treatment that chiropractors use to help our muscles function better, Applied Kinesiology, is also available in a simplified home version for everyday people to help reduce pain and stress levels. Small studies have shown that Applied Kinesiology is beneficial, though most medical doctors consider it highly suspect. I'm not making any claims about the health benefits of specialized kinesiology, but from personal experience, I know it has been crucial in giving me tools to reduce my stress and pain as well as helping me keep a level emotional state. I think being in less stress and pain is likely to be beneficial to my health in the long run, but that's just my opinion.

In case this topic has you rolling your eyes, I understand. Before I got sick, I had never heard of specialized kinesiology, but if I had I would have laughed at people who tried it. I was so closed-minded and intolerant that I probably would have thought of them as pathetic losers. Talk about having to eat crow. Here's how much I value it now: if I had no other tool to keep calm, I could live a comfortable life with only specialized kinesiology. This is not the best match for cerebral types who live life in their heads, since they are not connected enough to their bodies to tune into and recognize the changes. For them, I'd recommend beginning with Resistance Flexibility Strength Training (RFST.) You don't need to feel any connection to your body to realize the benefits you get from RFST.

Rather, I think of specialized kinesiology as being a perfect tool for people who are *overly* connected to their body; the highly sensitive types who are constantly struggling with strong body sensations, whether that's physical pain or emotional ups-and-downs.

An Easy Demonstration with the Five Elements

Follow along with this simple demonstration, and I'll explain how you can use it at home. Close your eyes for a moment and connect with a spot where you feel pain in your body. How painful is it on a scale of 0 to 10? Write that number down. Next think about the most emotionally-charged situation that is currently troubling you. How strongly are you impacted by it on a scale of 0 to 10? Write that down too. It's important to write these numbers down because we tend to forget how we were feeling once we start feeling better.

Five Elements Exercises

Next, use the diagrams on the next few pages to do the following five exercises. Repeat each movement three times, paying attention to the sensations in your body as you engage your muscles. The idea behind these exercises is that they shift energy in the body and allow the body to move out of fight or flight so we can better access our prefrontal cortex. You might notice that it's hard or a little uncomfortable to make one or more of the movements at first, yet it eases up as you go through the exercises. That is allowing energy to move in areas it might not normally go.

I find these types of movements, which are based on muscle tests that chiropractors use, are helpful for reducing pain in specific areas, such as the back, even if I don't have time to do all five of these exercises. You might want to memorize your favorites so that you can use them as needed.

BLADDER :: WATER
MERIDIAN   ELEMENT

SACROSPINALIS

Look over your left shoulder. Move your left shoulder forward in the direction of the arrow and then back to the starting position three times. Remember to breathe normally. Repeat on your right side.

LUNG :: METAL

MERIDIAN · ELEMENT

ANTERIOR SERRATUS

Bring your right arm above your head. Extend your right shoulder forward. Move your hand up and down like you are shaking hands with a giant three times. Repeat on your left side.

STOMACH :: EARTH
MERIDIAN   ELEMENT

PECTORALIS MAJOR
CLAVICULAR

Bring your right hand, thumb down, out in front of you at the midline of your body, shoulder height. Bring it down at a 45-degree angle towards your right hip as if you are swimming. Return to the starting point and repeat two more times. Repeat on your left side.

HEART :: FIRE

MERIDIAN   ELEMENT

SUBSCAPULARIS

Bring your left arm up, elbow at shoulder height and hand down, like a scarecrow. Bring your hand up while keeping your elbow in place. Return to starting and repeat two more times. Repeat on your right side.

LIVER :: WOOD

MERIDIAN   ELEMENT

RHOMBOIDS

Bring your elbows to your waist. Squeeze your shoulder blades together firmly towards your spine. Now move your left elbow away from your body and rotate your elbow up to be in line with shoulder level. Return to starting and repeat two more times. Repeat on your right side.

Noticing Your Body

Once you do these five exercises, be sure to check in with the pain in your body. Now how painful is that spot on a scale of 0 to 10? Did you get some relief? Has anything shifted for you emotionally on a scale of 0 to 10? These exercises are useful after a hard day's work to help shed the tension of the day, or in the morning if you dread going to work. You might try them on your kids before school or homework. These muscle movements are adapted from *Touch for Health: The Complete Edition,* used with Matthew Thie's permission. If you find them helpful, imagine what movements specifically targeted to your own body's needs could do.

ESR with K27 Points

Another helpful exercise for stress relief is to rate your pain and emotional distress on a scale of 0 to 10 and write that down. Next, follow the diagram on the next page. Place the thumb and index finger of one hand on your forehead at the points marked ESR (which stands for Emotional Stress Release) in the diagram below. Take the other hand and place your thumb and index finger in the notches below your collarbones marked as K27. These are at the end of the kidney meridian. If you're finding the right notches, they'll likely have tender bumps. Take a deep breath and relax. Tell yourself that you're safe and that all is well. Hold for about ten breaths or until you have the urge to sigh.

ESR with K27: Hold the ESR points with your thumb and index finger of one hand. Hold the K27 points with your thumb and index finger of your other hand. Close your eyes and breathe slowly, in for four counts and out for four counts. Keep on until you notice that you give a deep sigh.

Holding Points

Rate your pain and emotional distress again. Have they improved? This combination of points is from PanHarmonic Healing (PHH) and I've found it incredibly helpful for me to reset to calm. This is just a small taste of PHH. There is much more that PHH can do to help us be more comfortable in our bodies.

Holding points on the body is an example of specialized kinesiology. These examples can be used to help lighten your mood, lessen your pain levels, and increase your energy. I do some sort of kinesiology on myself every day. A side benefit of specialized kinesiology has been that as I get the emotional holding patterns out of the way, I feel more connected to my soul and aligned with my higher power. I've been told that some recovering addicts/alcoholics find it helpful to use specialized kinesiology as part of their toolkit for maintaining their sobriety. Specialized kinesiology may be helpful for other issues. Recent studies have shown that some people with borderline personality disorder may be misdiagnosed and instead need treatment for PTSD. Studies also show that children who are diagnosed with depression or ADHD could really be suffering from trauma. Perhaps this is why specialized kinesiology is of benefit, since I've found it helps release emotional trauma.

Can You Sense an Argument?

Have you ever felt the impact from the dark cloud of an argument when walking into a room? Our bodies generate a weak electromagnetic signal when we think or feel or move. That weak electromagnetic signal is a part of non-verbal communication. Some people are very sensitive to this type of communication, particularly introverts. This electromagnetic signal extends around our bodies. Thoughts are energy, emotions are energy. The stronger the thoughts and emotions, the more energy they generate. Our beliefs about ourselves impact our bodies, and others' beliefs and energies impact us as well.

Healthy Emotional Etiquette

When we interact with people, even indirectly, our mirror neurons are engaged. We get a taste of their emotional state. Have you ever had a conversation with someone where you vent about a problem and feel better afterwards? You were discharging emotional energy. Have you ever had a conversation with someone where they vent about a problem and you feel terrible afterwards? They discharged their emotional energy onto you. It takes a skilled, mindful listener to create a safe space for someone to vent while not taking on the negative energy themselves. Some people never learn how to process their emotions; they look to other people to discharge on. It's important that our friends learn how to reciprocate, whether they are introverts or extroverts.

Part of my definition of introverts is that they are people who, often unknowingly, take on the unconscious concerns and emotions in the form of energy of other people. Part of my definition of extroverts is that they are people who can unknowingly hand off some of their concerns and emotions in the form of energy onto other people. An awareness of this issue is vital to keep us in good health. If we are sick, we need to protect ourselves from people who won't stop handing off energy without reciprocating. They may be unaware of the effect they have on introverts, but that makes them no less difficult to be around. Introverts also need to learn how to shield themselves from the energy drain so that they can be comfortable around others. Extreme introversion or extroversion is not healthy—we all need balance in our lives. Our tendency is often hardwired in us as a reaction to early childhood trauma. We'd do best to be flexible--situationally able to accommodate the need for introversion to recharge and extroversion to succeed in a business meeting.

Developing Boundaries

People with illnesses like fibromyalgia and chronic fatigue tend not to have boundaries. This is because in their childhood they constantly took the emotional temperature of their environment to stay safe. They looked to the outside at other people's emotional state rather than to their own emotional state for guidance. The same thing holds true for them in adulthood because it's an unconscious process. After a lifetime of giving, this can lead to becoming ill. Those who are sick often have surrounded themselves with family or friends who do not reciprocate or who keep them in a state of fear so they don't have to deal with their own fear.

Touch for Health, Brain Gym ® / Edu-K and PanHarmonic Healing are types of specialized kinesiology that can be invaluable in unlocking emotions and trauma stored in the body. These are all offshoots of Applied Kinesiology. Some people can feel energy moving in their body and some people can't, but most come away from a session with a sense of relaxation and catharsis, reduced pain and an increased sense of well-being.

Dissociating

When I first started working with a kinesiologist, I used to get very sleepy when some of the acupressure points were held. This sleepiness is a form of dissociating just like what can happen when we are first learning to Focus (see Chapter 20 for more information about Focusing.) I worked on becoming more present in the sessions over time, trying to stay with the sensation rather than caving into the sleepiness. I think of specialized kinesiology as a tool just like in Focusing, because after a while, I could choose to work on the emotional pain a little at a time until I got comfortable feeling almost any emotion. At first, I was so shut down that there were certain emotions I couldn't feel at all, even if I tried. Over time, though, I could learn how to pay attention to the sensations, however fleeting they were. Eventually those sensations lasted longer, until I could allow them in. After a long time, I could allow them to flow. There is nothing like the feeling of being rid of something that you've been holding for a long time. It's liberating. I practiced on myself every day to try to keep the momentum up and to learn how to be okay with whatever message my body was trying to give me.

Applied Kinesiology

Applied Kinesiology was created when a chiropractor, Dr. George Goodheart, started exploring the overlap between Traditional Chinese Medicine and the forty-two muscle tests that chiropractors use. As chiropractors began using Applied Kinesiology on patients, their patients learned bits and pieces and began to try to use it on themselves. One chiropractor who studied with Goodheart, Dr. John Thie, developed it into a lay process for regular people to be able to use for themselves and their families. He wrote a manual called *Touch for Health* and developed trainings so that anyone could learn how to release emotions for oneself, friends and family in a way to help support health and wellness in-between doctor and chiropractor visits.

The *Touch for Health* manual explains how the pain we feel in one muscle is often because its partner (called the opposing muscle) is underactive. The first muscle does too much of the opposing muscle's work for it. If we can get the energy to flow to the muscle that is not being used, it reduces the strain on the muscle that is causing the pain. The problem is that we tend to have patterns of muscle use that we can trace back to our childhood. For example, if we weren't allowed to express our anger, the muscles in the liver and gallbladder meridians might not be firing well. If we weren't allowed to express our fear, the muscles connected to the kidney and bladder meridians might not be working correctly. If fear was the only emotion we were allowed to express, the kidney and bladder meridians may be overused. Touch for Health can help us release those patterns and start developing healthier new ones.

Touch for Health Sessions

A Touch for Health session educates you about how to use this system for yourself. You create a session goal, which is a positive affirmation for yourself. You notice the level of physical and emotional pain you're in. The instructor uses a fourteen, twenty-eight or forty-two muscle test which is based on the forty-two-muscle test that chiropractors use to see which meridians are blocked. They then use Traditional Chinese Medicine points and other techniques to unblock the meridians. Once the energy is flowing again, they check with you to see if the pain is gone. It often is. If not, they use additional techniques from the Touch for Health manual to help reduce it further. Then they retest the muscles, which should be firing normally, and work on any additional areas if they are still not firing well. You're given some everyday techniques to help increase your comfort. You leave feeling refreshed, calmer and in less pain. Touch for Health sessions are particularly helpful using a technique called a Reactive Muscle Balance. This type of balance assists in resetting spasming muscles. It's also effective in helping other types of pain.

When I wanted to learn how to help spread the word about specialized kinesiology, I started by learning Touch for Health. It has such strong connections to chiropractic that it will seem the most familiar to people. It also has the most comprehensive instruction manual I've ever seen. By tuning in regularly to our bodies, we are more aware when we need to see a health professional, allowing us to get help sooner.

Storing Emotions

As mentioned earlier, the mind is incredibly efficient, storing specific emotions along specific muscles and organs so they are easy to find again and learn from later until they are accepted, processed and released. Specialized kinesiologists can help us access these pathways through the training that they have had. We learn how to process and release emotions through use of acupressure and other tools.

Brain Gym ®

A very helpful offshoot of Touch for Health is called Brain Gym ®. Brain Gym ® is a part of Breakthroughs International. Brain Gym ® helps synchronize the body to allow learning. Brain Gym ® was developed by an educational professional, Paul Dennison, who was a Touch for Health instructor. He had learning disabilities, and developed a program to help himself, which in turn has helped thousands of others to learn more easily. Brain Gym ® has been used by teachers since 1986 to help our children use their eyes better, pay attention in class, and otherwise wake up the brain to learn without stress or strain. Adults can be helped by Brain Gym ® too. They typically have lots of behavior patterns developed during childhood which no longer serve them, yet are stuck in place. Brain Gym ® can help adults shed the past and move forward in order to achieve our life goals. They've been vitally important to my healing.

PanHarmonic Healing

As I mentioned earlier, I've also gotten a lot of help from a type of specialized kinesiology called PanHarmonic Healing, developed by Santa Barbara chiropractor Dr. Valerie Girard. I've been going to weekly sessions with a specialized kinesiologist, Julie Newendorp, for the last three years, who was trained in part by Dr. Girard. Once I got to a certain point in my work with Julie, she suggested I take Dr. Girard's training so I could help myself between sessions. It has been a game changer. I've found it easy to learn how to use this system to have tools whenever uncomfortable feelings come up. Of all the types of specialized kinesiology I've tried, it's the one I find easiest to work on myself with. It has a comprehensive system to deal with a lot of emotional energies. Other kinesiologies do wonderful things for me too, but require a practitioner for me to get the best from them.

Expressing Feelings

Going to psychotherapy in my twenties was helpful, but it unintentionally gave me tools to only deal with the mind. I started rationalizing away my feelings, rather than tuning into them. I explained away others' hurtful actions, so that my empathy was only for other people, which meant my own feelings were never honored. Now I know I have to express my feelings and once they're heard and acknowledged, even if it's only within myself, they can change. They are only set in stone when they're not expressed.

A specialized kinesiology session consists of taking stock of what's been happening and what emotions have come up during the week. You might take notes during the week of what you want to accomplish in a session (what major events happened to you that week, how you felt about them, how your life goals are going, and anything important that came up during psychotherapy) and discuss this with your kinesiologist when you first start the session. Your own body is the guide. It has priorities on what holdings it needs to release and which order it wants to release them in. Your body heals itself.

The practitioner is only there to help you access its wisdom until you learn enough to access its wisdom on your own. At the start of a session, the client sits and discusses their goals for the session. Once that's established, the practitioner begins muscle testing to see where nerve energy is blocked. The practitioner can work with the client standing up or with the client lying on a massage table. The client is always fully clothed and in charge of how the session proceeds.

Combining Kinesiologies

Any of these kinesiologies are great on their own, however a combination session offering multiple modalities lets you go in whichever direction your body needs. For example, a combination of Touch for Health, Brain Gym ® and PanHarmonic Healing lets the kinesiologist see where energy is blocked in the body, allows old patterns to be released, and healthy new ones to be integrated. Often the process releases something from the present which is linked to something in the past. The client leaves the session with a sense of calm, and new tool for how to better handle their emotions. It's easy from the start to quickly learn tools to clear any shock or trauma from interacting with the world.

Tools to Feel Safe

For the lucky ones who can feel energy moving, these sessions give a feeling of safety. They can feel energy draining away as a cold or warm feeling, as numbness or tingling, or as muscle twitches, which in my experience is a part of the emotion getting processed. Even if they can't feel the energy moving, once the points are released, the emotion stops. It might bring on a strong emotion at first while the points are being held, but the client is in control of that because they set the pace of the session. Knowing the feeling goes away once the release is completed can encourage them to hang in there, both during sessions with their kinesiologist as well as with work they do on themselves at home.

Developing Personal Power

We often start to panic when we have a bad feeling. Typically, we shut down the connection to our body and try to think about or do something else, often to the point of reaching for a bottle or a pill. If we don't like being out of control, we might shrink our life smaller until finally we are afraid to try anything.

Once I started seeing a specialized kinesiologist and learning tools for home use, my new pattern was to work on myself every day whenever bad feelings came up. Using these tools left me with a feeling of calm, and helped me gain a bit of personal power to be able to reset my old patterns.

Specialized kinesiology gives us invaluable tools to know when we're experiencing our own emotions and when we're being influenced by other's emotions, as well as helping us to clear emotions. We all have emotions 24/7--they don't just happen at the kinesiologist's office. Learning these techniques can allow us to stop reliving the past and start enjoying our lives to the fullest.

We Are All More Interconnected Than We Know

As I mentioned earlier, introverts become very good at picking up others' emotional states to stay safe. As you learn specialized kinesiology and how to clear your energy, you'll likely become more aware of what is impacting your body. The next time you're feeling fine one minute and the next minute you're in throbbing pain, you'll have the tools to know if it's your emotion or if you've picked up someone else's energy.

I've found we are more vulnerable to getting sick when we are around other people who are projecting negative energy. We can also feel more pain around some people's energy too. If someone is in pain or crisis, an empath picks up that energy and it is reflected in the empath's body. My kinesiologist encouraged me to learn more about the body's energy systems, including how to heal auras and how to strengthen one's hara. The hara is the area of the belly that Japanese martial arts were developed to strengthen. It's connecting to the energy from the gut brain which is connected to chi beyond us. If you've ever seen a demonstration where black belt masters can make themselves too heavy to lift, this is the energy they draw from.

The Body's Energy System

I noticed that sometimes after being around certain people I'd come away feeling physically terrible. Sometimes it'd be my back or neck going out, sometimes it'd be a sense of general fatigue. Occasionally, if I was eating a meal with a person who seemed upset or irritable, I'd get sick immediately. For example, one time I had a coughing fit and huge reaction to a food that normally doesn't affect me. Within a minute my health took a nosedive, beyond what could be explained by how fast germs multiply. Every time that happened, during my next balance, my kinesiologist would test my aura and it'd be ripped open. The skeptic in me got all the proof I needed because I don't make enough endorphins to hide pain. I am overly sensitive to all sensations, so I could feel it as she re-knit my aura each time.

Re-knitting the Aura

A practitioner re-knits an aura by moving their hands over the energy field between 1-3 inches away from the client's body and muscle testing to make sure the aura is now strong again. Re-knitting made me aware of having a wound which I hadn't know existed. It gave me the soothing feeling that the equivalent of ointment and a Band-Aid had been put on that wound. I felt a sensation of there being some boundary to me beyond my body that started to get filled up again each time it got re-knit. This was the first time I realized that part of what I thought of as being sick was really about that energy layer being breached. It made me realize I needed to learn more about auras and other levels of our energy body.

Connecting to the Field

For most people, taking classes in these specialized kinesiologies or going to sessions to process pain or emotions will be all they ever want to accomplish and all they ever need to have a happier, healthier life. For those on a spiritual path, though, it seems specialized kinesiology can connect us to a deeper wisdom and a higher path. Much of what causes pain in this world is caused by people overly invested in their ego-selves, who have no skills to cope with strong emotion. That describes me, before I started to heal. I have found that specialized kinesiology allows me to connect to my higher self. It allows the ego-self to be set aside, at least for the space of a session, to undo whatever negative programming from the past is currently up for healing, to reset to calm, and tap into a greater good and one's highest life direction. If you've heard of or seen the popular movie *The Secret,* which teaches about the law of attraction, the emotional clearing taught in PanHarmonic Healing can be used to assist people to stay in touch with divine will by helping keep the ego in check. In this way, the right brain can stay connected to that which is greater than us. People can use it to allow themselves to reset when they are upset, so they remain in a higher level of thinking and connection.

The Hundred Monkey Principle

In much the same way as the hundred-monkey principle works (that once a hundred monkeys on one side of an island learn a skill, the monkeys on the other side of the island with no contact also develop the skill) there appears to be a deeper interconnectedness to consciousness than our culture currently recognizes. It is said that the more people there are on a spiritual path, the more awake and aware the cultures of our planet will be. To use the term as Lynne McTaggart uses in her book *The Field*, it is thought that the development of these kinesiologies could be meant for that purpose. I teach Touch for Health and PanHarmonic Healing levels 1 & 2. The contact information for my teachers and my kinesiologists are in the action steps listed below. I hope I'm a good example of how much help they are with supporting traumatized people to heal.

Has the Author Lost Her Mind?

I'm sure some of you are wondering this, so I'll address it directly. Here was my logic: I spent the first forty-two years of my life asleep, and it led to autoimmune disease. As I began to wake up and question my thoughts, my beliefs and my life, I realized that I could not control my feelings and that denying my feelings had made me sick. I'd run my life completely through my mind, that is to say, my ego-self, and it had led me to illness. It seemed clear to me that some of my beliefs had to be wrong, as well as some of my thoughts and patterns of behavior. When I had a specialized kinesiology session, I could go beyond anxiety and fear, beyond anger, to feel interconnected and whole. The conscious mind is only about five percent of our whole brain. There is so much said in our culture about listening to our gut and following our intuition. It seems that our intuition is connected to our unconscious; to the greater part of our mind and body. It also seems to be interconnected in some way to others and to that which some call God or The Universe. Why not give that gut instinct a chance to guide me, I reasoned? Certainly, my tiny rational mind had screwed up royally. My programming was faulty. I was overly fearful about everything. My body was exhausted. Perhaps there was a better guidance system on board that I could tap into while I was in that connected state? And so, I began to take baby steps into that reality. It was daunting, because surrendering control when one has been captain of one's ship for a lifetime feels at times like an extremely bad idea. And yet, over time, I could see that it led me to a healthier state. To empathy for myself when needed and empathy toward others when needed. To undoing a lifetime of self-sabotaging patterns and developing healthy self-love. Away from inflammatory thought spirals and emotional shipwrecks and towards clarity. More able for my rational mind to be a calm parenting influence on my scared inner children and more able to lead those inner children to reconnect and heal. And that's why I recommend specialized kinesiology to those on a spiritual path.

Additional techniques

I have also found something called Ask and Receive as well as Emotional Freedom Technique (EFT) helpful in supporting trauma release. You can find more about these techniques below.

Action steps:
Easy:

Try Ask and Receive at askandreceive.org

Learn more about EFT at thetappingsolution.com, or read Nick Ortner's book *The Tapping Solution: A Revolutionary Method for Stress-Free Living* or Jack Canfield's *Tapping into Ultimate Success.*

If you're open to it, keep up a positive frame of mind with Notes from the Universe. They are free. Sign up at tut.com.

Moderate:

Try specialized kinesiology. You can find a nearby instructor at touchforhealth.us or for Brain Gym ® at breakthroughsinternation.org. There are lots of caring, empathetic instructors available to help you and they are closer than you think.

Matthew Thie is the son of John Thie and is the co-author of the *Touch for Health: Complete Edition* manual. He offers group classes in Los Angeles and around the world. He's a wonderful instructor. You can find him at Touch4health.com.

If you are looking for a Touch for Health reactive muscle balance, look for someone who is certified as Touch for Health Proficient, a Touch for Health instructor or consultant. These three types of Touch for Health practitioners are certified as in giving a 42-muscle balance, which I've found to be a necessary part of a reactive muscle balance. It requires a double session to do this type of balance, but I've found it to be well worth it.

Sign up for a class in PanHarmonic Healing. You can look at my website, rightbrainuniversity.com, to see when I offer classes or contact Valerie Girard at panharmonic.com.

Julie Newendorp is the founder and president of the Nurturing

Parent Center. She's a gifted healer and a great resource for us all. Her website is nurturingparentcenter.com.

Harder:

Sign up for an online class with my aura and hara teacher, Talitha Wall, at Lionsgate School at lionsgateschool.com.

I was first introduced to specialized kinesiology by a talk I saw Paula Oleska give at Omega Institute. I've enjoyed working with Paula. Her website is naturalintelligencesystems.com.

Thursday:

Develop Parasympathetic Breathing, Exercise, Vision and Thoughts

Chapter 16
Breath Is More Than Just Getting Air Into Us

Breath is Also About How We Breathe—Using the Parasympathetic vs. Sympathetic Nervous Systems

As I mentioned in Chapter 3, our autonomic nervous system (ANS) is divided into three types: sympathetic (SNS), parasympathetic (PNS) and enteric (ENS). The ANS regulates all our internal organs and glands unconsciously. That means that the right brain is in charge of processing it, which is yet another reason we need a well-developed right brain.

Sympathetic = Fight or Flight = Inflammatory

I would have thought the sympathetic nervous systems, the SNS, would be our best friend because the name reminds me of sympathy, but this is the pathway that causes inflammation. It produces the fight-or-flight response to help keep us alive in times of immediate danger, and is also the system that causes the problem with chronic stress.

Another important duty of the SNS is to stay active at a low level to help maintain a constant immune response in our bodies to support life.

Breathing Stressed Means Feeling Stressed

When we breathe through our mouths we are inadvertently signaling our bodies that there may be danger. The next time you feel angry or stressed, notice if you are breathing through your mouth. If so, bring your breath back to breathing calmly through your nose. This is why yoga and meditation both primarily use nose breathing.

The Parasympathetic Nervous System is Calming

The parasympathetic nervous system (PNS), the liver, the kidneys and the brain also work with the SNS to help us maintain a constant state to support life. The PNS is calming and reduces inflammation. It's in charge whenever we rest or digest. When we breathe through our noses we feel calmer because we are activating the PNS.

Breathing Styles are Passed Down From Parents to Children

Stressed parents pass down their stressed breathing habits to their children as children mimic their parents' behavior. How we breathe can either activate our SNS or PNS. For long term health, we want our breathing to keep us in a steady, calming, healthy non-inflammatory state.

We want to breathe in a way that keeps our PNS active as much as possible. Our body knows how to immediately shift to SNS in a stressful situation. Back when I got migraines frequently, I used to catch myself "not breathing enough." I thought maybe I was oxygen-deprived, and perhaps that's why I kept getting so many migraines, so I'd start speeding up my breathing. I learned the hard way that breathing is not supposed to be under conscious control. I was accidentally increasing the amount of inflammation in my sinuses and bronchia.

Making the Switch from Mouth to Nose Breathing

The SNS can take care of itself, but many of us need to learn how to activate PNS breathing. This goes beyond simply breathing through your nose whenever possible. I had no idea that this could be a stressful process until I tried it. For people like me who are more emotional and anxious, it can be a big transition to learn how to switch over. If you want to try this, I'd suggest going slow. Keep it positive by thanking yourself for trying to change rather than getting frustrated if it's not easy for you. Realize your breathing does not have to change overnight or even in a month or two. You are heading toward better health simply by trying to learn this.

Children Who Have Trouble With Nose Breathing

Dental decay caused by mouth breathing at night is a common problem with kids and adults who have nasal congestion. We can reduce our children's risk of cavities as well as our own by making sure we all can breathe through our noses at night.

When Breathing Style and Nutritional Issues Meet

My younger son had several instances of enlarged adenoids and tonsils. His ENT doctor wanted to operate on his enlarged adenoids, which were blocking his breathing, but I wanted to look for nutritional alternatives because I remembered something I'd read about in *Let's Get Well* by nutritionist Adelle Davis.

Her books need to be updated, but it's possible to cherry pick great health tips from them. Her advice for this enlarged tissue was to mix the following until dissolved in a glass of warm water: 1000 mg powdered vitamin C, 200 mg B5 and 10 mg of B6. Her suggested dosage – "One teaspoon of this mixture given every two to three hours around the clock." Every day I gave my younger son one teaspoon of this mixture in the morning and one in the afternoon. He was not fond of it, but could tolerate it. He was breathing more easily every week. This formula isn't meant to be a substitute for a good, well-balanced diet, and it isn't meant to be used daily, but rather when we see an acute sore throat causing tonsil or adenoid swelling. According to Davis, some families have a high need for vitamin B5, pantothenic acid, and I've certainly found that to be true for mine.

After three months, I took my son back to be checked by the ENT. The doctor took one look and called off the surgery. He didn't even need a new scan because my son's adenoids looked totally normal.

This mixture has proven to be so important that I keep a stockpile in dry form in the cupboard ready to mix with water in the middle of the night if needed. I make a big batch of it: 50,000 mg of vitamin C, 10,000 mg of B5, and 500 mg vitamin B6 (that is 1 capsule of powdered 500 mg B6, 20 capsules of 500mg B5 and 100 capsules of powdered 500 mg vitamin C).

About a year later, my younger son had a severe sore throat and his tonsils puffed up so far into his mouth that he looked like a cottonmouth snake. My ex-husband thought he needed emergency room treatment and to have his tonsils removed. Instead I pulled out that formula again and gave it to my son every hour. Within three hours his tonsils had shrunk about halfway back to normal. I continued giving my son the mixture until his tonsils were back to normal size. Be sure to get your doctor or nutritionist's okay before trying this on your child. (My thanks to the Adelle Davis Foundation for allowing use. More info about the foundation in this chapter's action steps.)

Issues with Asthma, Allergies and Snoring
On my journey, I came across the Buteyko breathing method developed by a Russian scientist, Constantin Buteyko.

Buteyko realized that our body needs a higher concentration of carbon dioxide than what is currently in our atmosphere. If we over-breathe (take in too much air) such as when we have a cold, cough a lot, or are emotionally stressed, our body will create inflammation around our airways to prevent loss of carbon dioxide.

Over-breathing Can Set up a Cycle of Inflammation, Asthma and/or Allergies
This means people who are emotionally stressed tend toward asthma. Buteyko believed the same pathway happens with allergies as well, where over-breathing leads to inflammation which is often connected to a specific allergen as an emotional trigger. All of this is played out on a completely unconscious level.

The Buteyko Method has had a great deal of success in helping severe asthmatics reduce or even eliminate their need for rescue inhalers. My favorite Buteyko Method trainer is Tess Graham, the mother of children with chronic asthma who were cured through breath retraining. Helping others has become her life's mission, and she's a lovely human being. Her program is based on and authorized by the late Professor Constantine Buteyko. Tess is an Australian-based physiotherapist with a degree in the Buteyko Breathing Method direct from Moscow, and a clinical practice in breath retraining. She has two books, *Relief from Snoring and Sleep Apnea*, and *Relief from Anxiety and Panic* as well as an online program.

There's a breath retraining program in Woodstock, NY that I struggled with because it moved a bit too fast for me. If you remember to follow your gut instincts in making a choice, I'm sure you'll do well with either program. Contact details for both are in the action steps.

Switching to Nose Breathing at Night

My experience has taught me that dealing with underlying emotional issues can lead to a reduction in the inflammation in my airways. Switching from mouth breathing to nose breathing, so that the parasympathetic nervous system is more active, helps to calm things down.

I was a mouth breather from childhood, but it turns out even I could change. It's easiest to transition first during the day to breathing through the nose. People may have emotional issues with this transition. I sure did. Clients are encouraged to breathe less, which can feel suffocating at first if they try too hard. I found it helped to take it very slowly. I thought of each breath through the nose as a victory and any time I reverted to mouth-breathing, I was patient and supportive of how hard it is to change.

After a certain point with the NY Buteyko method, they recommend a small piece of scotch tape over the mouth as a reminder not to mouth-breathe at night. Putting tape on my mouth made me feel panicky, but going to sleep with my hand on my lips was a good enough reminder for easing into it slowly. Especially for people who have had bronchitis to the point where they can barely breathe at night, any restriction at night can bring up that feeling of suffocation.

Now the only time I mouth breathe is when I have a cold, which I rarely have. I have gone from needing antibiotics six to eight times a year to not having been on antibiotics in years. For the past five years, I've been able to ward off most illnesses at the start with hydrogen peroxide in my ears as soon as I feel something coming on. I wouldn't recommend this if you tend to get ear infections, but for me, it's been a huge help to keep the lymph nodes in the neck clear and functioning.

Breathing and Fascia

Many of us have fascial restrictions through our rib cages and diaphragm. Usually this is a silent problem, although perhaps you feel breathless at times. You might have gotten checked out by your doctor without any problem being noted. You could have noticed you have a problem with how fully your rib cage and diaphragm can move if you try doing exercises lying down on one of those big fifty-inch diameter green balls. If you haven't, try lying down backwards on one. Do you feel breathless? How big a breath can you take? If you feel like you're unable to take a normal breath, it might be that your ribcage is bound up with fascia. When I first started working with my physical therapist, she had me work on a big green exercise ball. I was unable to move my ribs more than a half inch while lying on my back on it, so I couldn't breathe in properly while using it. If you notice the same problem, it's a good reason to seek out someone who does John Barnes MFR, a Rolfer, or a physical therapist.

Intercostal Release

I created and developed a process to be able to expand my ribs, so that my intercostal muscles would release. I would breathe in as far as I could, then hold my breath and try to make my ribcage

138

expand just a tiny bit more. I only practiced for 2 minutes a day. This is because how much in vs. out breath we take is a delicate process. It can impact the alkalinity of our blood and I wanted to be gentle on my system. Over time, I could stretch further and further. After about six months I felt and heard a huge popping sound within my ribcage, which was fascia releasing, though I didn't know it at the time. It didn't hurt at all. From that point on, it has allowed much more movement in my ribcage. I think the fascia constriction itself causes something we could call 'positional fear' or 'held fear' rather than fear caused in reaction to something happening currently in life. After releasing the fascia around the muscles in my ribcage and abdomen, freedom of movement has helped reduce emotional constriction. On average, I feel far less fear than I did before. Ask your doctor or physical therapist if you'd like to try this.

Action steps:
Easy:
Increase the amount of time you breathe through your nose. Notice how much you breathe through your mouth when you talk and try to use your nose to breathe instead.

If you catch yourself taking a deep breath without having exerted yourself, try to find the thoughts or feelings that triggered it. Release them through Focusing (see chapter 20) and/or PanHarmonic Healing.

Soothe your breathing and let it calm back down.

Moderate:
If you have problems with allergies, asthma, snoring or sleep apnea read Tess Graham's books or try her program at breathability.com. The NY Buteyko Method can be found at breathingcenter.com.

Try the RFST stretching program, whether book or video, to help free up your ribcage. See thegeniusofflexibility.com.

The Adelle Davis Foundation offers new copies of her books in

Kindle format through Amazon. They may have new print copies available by the time you read this book. Her foundation continues her nutritional legacy with education and scholarships. You can learn more at adelledavisfoundation.org.

Harder:

Work one-on-one with someone who does John Barnes MFR at myofascialrelease.com, or with an RFST trainer at thegeniusofflexibility.com to target your ribcage.

Try working with someone like Jada Delaney, who does Transformational massage (jadadelaney.cmt@gmail.com) or someone who does Chinese Chi Ne Tsang abdominal massage.

Chapter 17
Improving How We Exercise

Nose Breathing for Better Fitness Levels

As suggested by Dr. Douillard in his book *Body Mind Sport*, I've found it to be helpful to start breathing through my nose when I exercise. Modifying breathing to the parasympathetic state has been shown to reduce our risk of injury, since fight, flight or freeze puts us into our highest state of muscle, tendon and ligament tension. It also improves endurance levels if you breathe through your nose rather than your mouth. Lastly, in my experience, it also reduces sinus and lung congestion. My mild asthma went away.

When I first started experimenting with nose breathing in my spin bike workouts at the gym, I could only nose breathe for about twenty seconds before being so exhausted I would have to resume mouth breathing. I couldn't imagine ever being able to make the change. But after a few months of transition and building endurance I could do the entire forty-five-minute workout while breathing through my nose. I felt better, fitter and stronger.

If this sounds interesting, I'd recommend getting a doctor's clearance first. I think it's easiest to make the transition slowly, starting with trying it as you're walking around throughout your day. Once that starts feeling normal, move on to exercise. When you begin to exercise, breathe through your nose. If you feel like you need to breathe through your mouth, slow down your pace to see if you can keep from mouth breathing.

It's been found that high-intensity aerobic exercise is beneficial for increasing fast-twitch muscle fiber. Fast-twitch muscle fibers fatigue quickly but are used in bursts of movements like jumping or sprinting. If all we do is jog, all we're building is our slow-twitch muscle fiber. Slow-twitch muscle fibers can work for a long time without getting tired. They are used for long-distance activities that require endurance. Fast-twitch muscle accounts for about half of our muscle mass. It's used for rapid movements like sprinting. Kids naturally keep their fast-twitch muscle in top tone because they don't pace themselves. Instead, they run til they're exhausted and then they stop until they catch their breath and then they go at top speed again. We can learn from what they do.

This type of workout works well no matter what level of fitness you are at. Warming up for 3 minutes, sprinting for 30 seconds at whatever method of exercise you've chosen, then recovering for 1 1/2 minutes by walking. Keep that up for eight sprints, then cool down for 2 minutes. If you're out of shape, modify the number of sprints you try. Just warm up, sprint once, then cool down if that is what you need to start. This type of exercise is beneficial for metabolism, especially as we age.

The Benefits of Interval Training and Distance Running

A study by Mayo Clinic researchers recently published in *Cell Metabolism* showed that activity levels within genes changed with interval training in ways that are believed to influence the ability of mitochondria to produce energy for muscle cells, as compared to moderate exercisers or weight lifters. The changes impacted 274 genes in the younger participants, compared with 170 genes in moderate exercisers and only 74 for the weight lifters, but in the older study participants, almost 400 genes worked differently, compared to 33 for weight lifters and only 19 for the moderate exercisers.

While interval sprints are helpful for metabolism and mitochondria, it's not been found to be particularly beneficial for the brain. A study published in the *Journal of Physiology* recently by researchers at the University of Jyvaskyla in Finland working with rats, showed that the most beneficial form of exercise for the brain is distance running. It's believed that sustained aerobic exercise produces more BDNF (brain-derived neurotrophic factor) which regulates neurogenesis, the formation of new brain neurons in the hippocampus. In studies with animals, exercise on running wheels or treadmills has been shown to double or triple the number of new neurons compared to the brains of animals that remain sedentary. News like that has me dusting off my running shoes for both interval training and distance running. I also have started using jump rope to do interval training and am seeing quick metabolic benefits. It's also myelinating the brain through repetitive movement, so it's a win-win.

Do you Really Hate to Exercise?

If you think you hate to exercise, you might be wrong. I used to hate it until I realized what I hated is how I thought about myself when I exercised. Maybe you hate how you feel about yourself when you exercise too, or maybe you talk negatively to yourself when you exercise. Maybe kids made fun of your sports ability when you were young. Other people can undermine and sabotage us about exercise. They might not like us changing, even if they seem to encourage it. Actions speak louder than words, though, so look at their actions. We might not have much control over how others talk to us, but we are always in control over how we talk to ourselves. It will take time before we get good at catching our thoughts. If we keep practicing trying to pay attention to them, we can succeed. Same thing with what people said to us when we were kids—it's possible to get rid of negative programming through meditation, specialized kinesiology and therapy. Try these methods out and see which helps you release it best.

Setting Boundaries

If you've got saboteurs in your life, set boundaries. Renegotiate your relationships. Are your friends supportive? When you want to join a gym or yoga studio or buy exercise equipment, do you get a lecture from your significant other about how frequently you need to use the membership or the equipment? That can make you associate the gym and the equipment with feeling shamed. Try to explain to them how that undermines the very thing they are concerned about, because who wants to replay the shame tape every time you exercise? Ask them for support rather than lectures—-maybe by giving you a high-five every time you go to the gym or getting a kiss every time you get off the exercise bike. Think of ideas specific to you that might help you build positive, loving associations with exercise. There's nothing like being one's own best friend and coach to get the best out of ourselves.

Action Steps:
Easy:

Start listening to how you talk to yourself about exercise. Change it up if you're talking negatively to yourself. Get your doctor's blessing and begin a modest exercise program if you aren't already physically active.

Moderate:

Read John Douillard's book, *Body, Mind, Sport*, which has a very helpful Ayurvedic slant on exercise and breathing.

Harder:

Work with an RFST trainer. It's helped my family and me to free muscles that were gummed up with fascia and retraining them to work properly, so we can exercise better. It's also dramatically helped improve scoliosis for my family members.

As I mentioned before, for people with Fibromyalgia, I would recommend working with Luca Cupery and Kaj Hoffman in Santa Barbara, both RFST trainers. For people with ME/CFS (what used to be called Chronic Fatigue Syndrome), a friend has been helped a great deal by working with Karen Mason at RFST in Santa Barbara. Their practices are not limited to fibromyalgia and ME/CFS, but they have special feel for it, thanks to specific guidance from Bob Cooley. More at thegeniusofflexibility.com.

Chapter 18
Vision Therapy

Seeing 3-D

I still remember the first time I saw in 3-D. I was forty-two years old and I'd just gotten my first pair of prism glasses. I got in the car and put them on for the drive home. I drove about three blocks before suddenly everything went from normal to looking like someone had pulled the tabs in a children's pop-up picture book. I swear, if no one had been behind me, I would have caused an accident. My eyes were on the trees and the buildings and all the incredible space between things. My foot forgot that it had a job to do. My jaw dropped open. I must've dropped down to ten miles an hour before it even registered that I'd slowed down.

Once an optometrist prescribes glasses like these, the visual changes won't stick without vision therapy. The brain is used to processing vision in a certain way and once it's acclimated to the prisms, it will revert to its old patterns. I went to a vision therapy session every week for a year. Each week, I learned a new developmental vision exercise and was given daily exercises to do. Vision therapy and prism glasses dramatically reduced my anxiety levels and almost eliminated my migraines. It can even be useful for people with 20/20 vision, because sometimes people waste a lot of brainpower on suppressing vision from one eye in order to have 20/20 vision. An optometrist with training in vision therapy can catch that and correct it.

Can You See in 3-D?

Have you ever gone to a 3-D movie and been unable to enjoy the special effects everyone is oohing and aahing over? According to optometrists, as many as twenty percent of the population might not be able to fully see in three dimensions. People (like me) often don't realize they have a issue, or that the problem is bigger than getting a headache at a 3-D movie: it can impact our academic ability as well as our driving ability. It can make us more likely to trip and fall, and it can make us terrible at sports or only able to excel in specific kinds of sports.

The hard work of visual processing was a migraine trigger for me. Literally not knowing where I was in space created anxiety, although I didn't realize what the cause of the anxiety was until after treatment. Once I had prism glasses and finished vision therapy, driving was no longer stressful. Even jogging and walking had been causing me tension, but not anymore. If you have anxiety issues, you might want to consider seeing a vision therapist.

Master those Primary Reflexes

Perfect 3-D vision requires mastery of three primary reflexes: the Landau, the Asymmetric Tonic Neck Reflex, and the Pavlov Orientation. As mentioned before, primary reflexes are patterns of movement that are programmed into our brain to help us develop in utero and beyond, but they should be progressively mastered and no longer active by the age of three. Trauma can reactivate primary reflexes at any time in life.

These three primary reflexes prime the brain both for seeing and processing visual information automatically. The ideal visual field is like the MasterCard symbol: if each eye's visual field is represented as a circle, then both eyes together should see two circles with a bit of an overlap. This allows for the easiest conversion into a three-dimensional image. Too much overlap creates problems for the brain to process, as does too little overlap or no overlap at all. Problems with the amount of overlap makes the brain process vision with the cortex as a double-check rather than processing automatically. This reduces how much ability we have for executive thought.

Visual processing takes 80% of our brain's energy, so it's critical that it is automatic. We have two types of visual systems that our brain automatically switches between: peripheral and central vision. This can be thought of as global vs. focal or seeing the world vs. reading a book. Ideal vision would mean that the eyes lead the brain rather than the brain leading the eyes. In an ideal world, we wouldn't stay in either global or focal for any length of time; instead we would shift between them naturally so as not to overwork any particular set of eye muscles.

Brain Compensations

When we don't master the three primary reflexes mentioned above, one strategy is for our brain to take the 2-D images from each eye and flip between them, so it can construct a guesstimate what 3-D is like. If we are flipping between 2-D images, we tend to hold our breath when moving rather than being able to move and breathe at the same time, because breath-holding reduces the amount of information to process. People with this issue are in a constant state of internal tension. Their baseline internal state is set to 'overwhelmed' and they don't even know it because it's all they've ever known. As stated above, they can't optimize the use of their cortex, since their cortex is being used to second guess their vision to keep them safe in the world.

They are likely to try to keep their head as steady as possible because it is so much harder to process data when there is a big change in the horizontal plane. People with this problem tend to be more cautious with movement, and they are less athletic and physically interactive with the world than they are capable of being.

As I mentioned earlier, even if we have mastered the primary reflexes, anyone who has been traumatized is likely to have reactivated primary reflexes, which can take away our automatic vision. These reflexes can be reintegrated using kinesiology, which would be of help in vision therapy.

These kinds of visual issues can cause problems in academics. People without automatic vision carry much more stress from their delayed processing capacity. They work harder for poorer results. It takes energy to sort out the information from our environment that our brain is taking in as we work on a task—energy that could be better used to get our schoolwork done faster, better and with less strain if only our vision was automatic.

You can get help with primary reflex integration through Julie Newendorp's Nurturing Parent Center, among other places. More details are listed at the end of this chapter in the action steps.

Why I Go to a Vision Therapist

I had always gone to regular eye doctors, all of whom gave me stronger and stronger prescriptions over the course of my life. Unfortunately, I had too little overlap for my brain to make 3-D images automatically, only I never knew it. Kids with ADHD have three times the rate of convergence insufficiency than their typically-developing peers. Eye issues like these are also more common in the autistic spectrum community. Fortunately, thanks to a friend, I came across the office of Dr. Mel Kaplan, the director of the Center for Visual Management in Tarrytown, NY. A doctor of optometry, Dr. Kaplan had worked as a clinical instructor of behavioral sciences at New York Medical College and has published a body of research on ambient lenses and their role in helping people who struggle with learning, emotional or autistic spectrum disorders. He's written two books about vision: *Seeing Through New Eyes*, and *The Secrets in Their Eyes: Transforming the Lives of People with Cognitive, Emotional, Learning or Movement Disabilities*.

Distance Convergence Insufficiency

Regular eye doctors recognize the problem of near point convergence and know how to correct it, but they do not treat the distance convergence issue because it mimics needing regular distance prescription lenses.

This is what distance convergence insufficiency looked like for me: imagine you go to a theater to see a play and after a half hour or so, your eyes tire and the images blur. If you stop struggling to focus, the image would double. You could think of it as having situational double vision, which was all I ever had known, so I thought it was normal.

When eye doctors increased the prescription, it just gave me headaches from eye strain. Yes, I could see better briefly while being tested, but since that wasn't the problem, the eye strain got continually worse. As the eye strain grew worse over the years, so did my anxiety levels until it was crippling me. As Dr. Kaplan explains in his book *Seeing Through New Eyes*, it was all connected.

Eye Strain or the Wrong Prescription?

By the time I was in my forties, I could only use my glasses for driving and even then, I would get headaches from the amount of correction that I had been given. I ended up with 20/200 vision. After working with Dr. Kaplan and his vision trainers, my vision improved until it ended up at 20/30 and my anxiety levels dropped significantly. For the first time, I could hold onto a train of thought or follow someone's logic in an argument and see where it broke down, all because I had more brain power freed up for executive thinking.

Too much time in either focal vision (using a computer or reading a book) or global vision (searching the distance for a predator) causes stress in our systems. It is contracting to our bodies because when specific muscles in our eyes are used for too long without a break, it leads to spasm in muscles in the neck, shoulders and back. Contraction at its extreme causes pain. In our culture, we tend to spend too much time in focal vision from an early age, particularly now with computer and phone screens, along with teaching children to read at younger and younger ages. Being able to shift between global and focal vision is calming. When we are standing in nature, drinking it in, seeing the whole and feeling a part of it, it feels peaceful and soothing. We can think of too much time spent locked in one type of vision as activating the sympathetic nervous system and being able to shift between focal and global every ten minutes or so as activating the parasympathetic nervous system.

Our Kids with 2-D Vision Need Help

We need a balance between the two systems, but our society and our schooling overemphasizes focal vision. As school work gets more difficult in second, fourth and seventh grade, kids with 2-D vision have a hard time keeping up. More kids are diagnosed at these times with learning disabilities, but most are not tested for primary reflex issues or convergence insufficiency. It's a lost opportunity to be helped by vision therapy or physical therapy and kinesiology to integrate their primary reflexes.

If kids were tested for having good 3-D vision, they could more easily reach their full potential. To understand what goes on with 2-D vision, think of the brain's potential output like a river. A big part of the river for someone who sees 2-D is being diverted towards making a 3-D approximation of the world. With so much of our cortex's energy diverted this way, there are fewer resources for academic thinking in these kids than for others who have automatic 3-D vision.

Imagine All Kids Living up to Academic Potential

Kids who are intelligent in other ways but who have this vision problem are not going to live up to their academic potential. They often go through their school years with the feeling of being stupid because they know they are capable of much more than they can produce. This carries over into adulthood.

Additionally, their brain is working so hard that it leads to them being overwhelmed. We all have emotional overreactions when there is too much data for our brains to process. The brain gets overloaded. It sends that overload to the amygdala, which reacts with strong emotion like anger or fear.

Have you ever had to focus on a visual problem, like reading an instruction booklet to assemble a new gadget, while at the same time facing auditory demands from children in need of attention? A prime example happens during the holiday season. Did you get frustrated? Sometimes parents can blow their top when under bombardment like this. It's an example of what happens when the brain gets overloaded.

The Effect of Stress on Vision

Stress can also reduce our ability to see clearly, as can strong emotion, like anger. For example, if our upper trapezius muscles are tight it can blur our vision. Both stress and anger can tighten the upper trapezius. Many people who can get by as children and young adults lose their visual processing ability as they age. They start falling asleep when they try to read because they no longer have enough energy.

This reduces our lifetime productivity and enjoyment. People give up on school or don't try to return to school when they are smart enough to succeed and only their vision is holding them back. The worst thing is that brilliant people might spend their lives feeling dumb, while the rest of us lose out on benefitting from their talents.

It is often the smartest babies who figure out how to cheat the primary reflex system instead of following the prescribed movements. Stressed babies don't complete the primary reflex system properly either.

Visual Imbalance Causes Emotional and Physical Tension

Vision therapy helped me process emotions. I was unaware how much emotional and physical tension my eyes were causing me. After I got prism glasses and did therapy, my emotional tension dropped dramatically. Prism glasses allowed me to see objects where they really were in space, so my brain didn't have to make corrections. Once I knew where I was located in the world better, I felt more comfortable and had less physical tension. I was then able to process more information because my brain wasn't so occupied with keeping me safe in the world. Now I know more immediately how I feel. Before vision therapy, I needed to think constantly so that I could figure out how I felt. My poor brain was like a hamster on a wheel—compelled to exercise to the point of exhaustion. It was much too busy trying to keep me physically and emotionally safe. What a relief to finally have some peace of mind.

Over the course of my life, I had become increasingly frozen by my visual processing issues. Since getting new glasses and doing vision therapy I have written a novel, two screenplays as well as this book, learned how to do public speaking, coped with divorce, downsizing, and a cross-country move. I credit Dr. Kaplan and his vision therapy for allowing me to be open to new ways of seeing and thinking.

Monovision Contacts Lenses and Glasses

Monovision contact lenses and glasses have become a popular option for presbyopia, but they compromise depth perception and intermediate vision. Depth perception is a critical skill. A further complication of monovision contact lenses is that the resulting visual changes can cause some areas of the brain and body to receive too much blood, while others get too little. The brain is still trying to create 3-D vision, which reduces the amount of capacity for executive function. Given how hard I've worked to attain 3-D vision, and that I've been told by a neurologist that my fibromyalgia symptoms are connected to an imbalance between hemispheres, I'd never use monovision products and can't recommend them to anyone.

Action Steps:
Easy:

For everyone, I'd suggest trying to increase the amount of global vision you get daily. Going to the beach or a walk in nature is a way of engaging your global vision. So is going outside and watching clouds pass by as you look for shapes in them. It's a vital part of reducing stress.

Moderate:

If you're having trouble with chronic anxiety, depression and health issues, *even if you have 20/20 vision,* you might want to give vision therapy a try. Look for someone through the College of Optometrists in Visual Development online at covd.org. Get prism glasses if needed and do vision training.

Learn Touch for Health to give you resources to reduce muscle tension—in particular, targeting the upper trapezius muscles helped both reduce chronic shoulder pain and improve my vision.

Harder:

Find someone who does Brain Gym ® and Books Neural Therapy, who can integrate primary reflexes. Julie Newendorp, founder of the Nurturing Parent Center in Santa Barbara, uses all three. It's a great support for vision therapy. You can reach Julie at julie@nurturingparentcenter.com.

You can find more info about Books Neural Therapy (BNT) and work with Dr. Books at drphyllisbooks.com.

You can find out more information on primary reflexes through Svetlana Masgutova's book *MNRI Dynamic and Postural Reflex Pattern Integration* available at masgutovamethod.com. She also has her own network of trained therapists to help with primary reflex integration.

Chapter 19
Rhythm and Timing Therapies

The Benefits of These Types of Therapies

One of the most important things our brain does is coordinate timing: timing between all the different parts of the brain with the organs, timing between the left and right sides of the body and brain, timing for the immune system, for digestion and most important, to keep us safe in the world of motion. Therapies that help develop this region have the added benefit of also improving impulse control.

Rhythm and timing therapies help develop synaptic connections with targeted exercises, ideally to a beat. They give the brain a chance to practice coordinating timing. Rhythm and timing therapies have been an important part of helping me recover from ADHD and its related anxiety and depression. The way the brain processes information is malleable. If you have any doubts, read the books *The Brain that Changes Itself* by Norman Doidge and *The Woman Who Changed Her Brain*, by Barbara Arrowsmith Young. I've gone a different route from Barbara Young's, but my route back to health as well as to grow beyond ADHD has been through stepping out of my old brain programming by reprogramming my brain. Bön/Buddhist meditation, yoga, MFR, RFST, therapy, vision therapy and specialized kinesiology have all been vital to the process.

Interactive Metronome

Another big help has been increasing my processing speed using Interactive Metronome (IM), a software program that uses a metronome beat to give the user feedback on how far off they are in attempting to keep time to a beat. Clients wear a trigger on their hand, use a floor trigger, or one in their shoe that provides feedback to the computer. This research-backed program grows synaptic connections as well as dendrites. Synapses and dendrites help neurons talk to each other. Movement while using IM lays down additional myelin onto the axonal portion of neurons. This helps signals travel up to five times faster than if a neuron has an incomplete myelin sheath. A strong myelin sheath also is protective to a neuron.

I got trained in Interactive Metronome to help a family member before realizing how much it could help me too. Using IM has helped me reduce my ADHD symptoms. I've had a lifelong problem with organization, distractibility, attention, procrastination, anxiety and depression. I had some success in the work world (I handled $70 million a year in import goods for a woman's clothing manufacturer) by putting all my brain power into my job. Once I had children, even as a stay at home mom, I couldn't cope with the chaos of organizing a household. I could barely keep my own head above water; having twins was beyond my ability. My anxiety and depression got worse and an autoimmune illness flared up, fed in part by the anxiety and sleeplessness. IM has been a big help to being able to function again.

What's Fired Together is Wired Together

The premise of IM is that what is fired together is wired together. When you repeat an experience over and over, the brain then learns to trigger the same neurons each time.

At first, the IM I did for myself helped me with reaction time and my ability to maintain a conversation. I was one of those people with such a meandering thought process that I would regularly lose my original train of thought. It was humiliating, so I kept my mouth shut more and more. IM helped clear up my thinking.

After I finished Vision Therapy, I still had problems with reversing a car in a straight line. It was especially important that I improve because the house I lived in at the time had a narrow and steep driveway bordered by high retaining walls. In the wintertime, the driveway got ice and snow on it regularly. I needed to back out with precision, since ice could make the tires slip towards the retaining walls. I did another round of IM, where I specifically targeted peripheral visual response to the metronome beat for my weak left eye/right brain combo. It was incredibly hard, because I basically almost couldn't do it. I had to ease my way in with some auditory input. Over time, it got easier and easier because I was growing synaptic connections that grew my ability to see peripherally. Now I'm able to reverse in a straight line with complete comfort and parallel parking has also dramatically improved.

The latest round of IM I did was about figuring out new ways to target what I think needs to be wired together better in my brain. One of the things I came up with is to do Interactive Metronome while filing bills. That means I'm growing my working memory (engaging the rules of filing) at the same time I'm practicing filing. I've been doing other working memory tasks and games while doing IM as well.

Because rhythm and timing is housed in the right prefrontal cortex and I know my right hemisphere is underdeveloped thanks to a neurologist, I am intentionally targeting the left side of my body to keep the beat and further develop the right hemisphere.

Right Brain University (RBU)

I founded Right Brain University to teach people tools to cope with emotions, spread the word about how to heal, and to help people improve the functioning of their brain.

I've developed a program through RBU to try to improve the brain more deeply than with Interactive Metronome (IM) alone. IM has been proved to make synapses and myelinate them. I got to wondering if the results could be improved by putting the body and brain into balance using specialized kinesiology before a session. If it worked, it could mean that we were getting a better *quality* of synaptic connections, not just an increased *quantity* of synaptic connections.

I test to see if a client has any retained primary reflexes that are preventing their brain from optimally functioning and clear that first. Then I go through looking for any meridians that have nerve energy blocks and clear them. I look for movement issues in the different layers of the brain. The cortex handles left-right movement, the midbrain handles up-down movement and the brain stem handles forward-backward movement. Any of these could be off, or a combination. I check whether the gait reflexes are automatic and whether the client has any stress associated with using his or her eyes and if there is any auditory intake stress.

It's still early days, but my first clients are having amazing success. One high school student who was struggling with the SAT Math prep test (completing only 40 out of 60 in timed tests and of those 40, little better than 50% were correct) did 11 sessions of RBU-IM and got an 800 on his Math SAT. Another high school tennis player wanted to improve his tennis game. He came away happy with his improved reaction time, but also with a newfound ability to study longer on school subjects that bored him. Before, despite being a good student, the most he could study was 20 minutes if he was bored. Afterwards, he reported that he could study 30-40 minutes on boring content. I plan to use this to help people who have been held back by their test-taking ability, as well as people who are looking to improve their visual processing speed, among others. By the way, as part of the IM treatment, I suggest asking one's doctor or nutritionist if it's okay to add omega-3 capsules high in DHA, as well as lecithin to the diet to help support production of myelin.

Yoga

A repetitive yoga practice like Core Power hot yoga or Svaroopa's restorative yoga also develop myelin in the body and brain. Bikram yoga is a good example of this too. With every movement, you are laying down myelin. Practicing the same routine two or three times a week is going to help keep neurons protected with myelin as well as challenge balance in a way that will maximize the brain's motor neuron development. Be sure to get your doctor's blessing before trying it.

Tibetan Bön/Buddhist Meditation

This type of meditation is sometimes called Tibetan Yoga. The outer Tsa-Lung uses a repetitive breath and movement pattern which also develops myelin in the body and brain over time. It is calming in its own right, but because of the repetitive movement it's also a myelin developer. It's much more than that, but for those looking to maximize myelin production, it's good to include.

Other ideas

Martial arts are another type of exercise that develops myelin because of repetitive movement. Japanese sword training, a part of Samurai training, is equally complex, precise, and repetitive. Think of anything you might do that contains an element of repetitive training and you can adapt it. Regular golf drills, tennis drills, and swimming drills all come to mind. These are powerful ways to keep the brain young.

Jump rope has become part of my new go-to routine. It's great for rhythm and timing. It develops a unique type of core strength—despite my hot yoga routine, I found it very hard and tiring at first. I started out doing interval training with it, jumping rope for thirty seconds and then resting and repeating for fifteen minutes. It wasn't easy because I wasn't coordinated enough. Over time, I've progressed to jumping rope for sixty seconds and in between sets holding a medicine ball while doing squats. I do six reps of jumping rope in fifteen minutes. I think it's great for helping to circulate lymph too. I like the fact that I enjoyed doing it as a kid, and after progressing at it I am doing well enough that I feel eager to do it rather than it feeling like a chore.

Action Steps:
Easy:

Read *The Brain that Changes Itself* by Norman Doidge and *The Woman Who Changed Her Brain*, by Barbara Arrowsmith Young.

Moderate:

Look for a repetitive movement class like yoga, martial arts or take your favorite sport and integrate a repetitive movement drill from it two to three times a week.

Buy a jump rope and get your doctor's blessing to use it. Go slow and be encouraging of your efforts.

Harder:

Try IM or its cheaper cousin Bal-A-Vis-X, a hand-eye coordination exercise program which develops rhythm and timing at a much slower pace than IM. Find an IM practitioner near you at interactivemetronome.com.

Find out more about Bal-A-Vis-X at bal-a-vis-x.com. It is designed to be used in school classrooms.

Consider vision therapy if you don't have perfect 3-D vision. The world should look like a children's picture pop-up book. If it doesn't, you might need help. Find a visual optometrist through the College of Optometrists in Visual Development online at covd.org.

You can find out more about my work at Right Brain University at rightbrainuniversity.com.

Chapter 20
Left-Brain Healing Therapies that Work

Therapy and Humanistic Psychology

It's a common human survival mechanism to separate from our feelings when we get traumatized. Even relatively minor things can be traumatic for young children, especially if they are highly sensitive. Traditional therapy is useful for giving us an understanding of our situation, but it's not uncommon that as much as psychoanalysis can help us, it can also end up giving us resources to further separate from our feelings. In my twenties and thirties, I certainly used the tools I learned in therapy this way. Understanding why other people were experiencing the world a certain way gave me an excuse to take their side over my own. Since emotions are a survival mechanism, we don't have that as an option. It's not about choosing sides. We must allow ourselves to experience emotions. Experiencing them doesn't mean acting on them. I've found that it's suppressing them that leads to a buildup and subsequent venting that make this seem to be a linked process, but it doesn't have to be.

In my experience, it's important to find a therapist who takes a holistic approach, who makes sure to stop you when you are expressing a feeling to ask where it is happening in your body, however annoying or threatening that might be to you, because in the long run, it is what will heal you. I remember being annoyed at my therapist at the time in Nyack, New York, Alan Levin, when he first introduced this to me. He kept asking me what I felt and where I felt it in my body. It seemed irrelevant at the time, and yet it was the key to getting well.

The cure that therapy provides can only really happen once we find someone with whom we feel safe enough to do the work of feeling those feelings.

Feeling Emotions Heals Us

Avoiding the feelings led me to the path of chronic illness. Letting myself feel the feelings is what made me well. There is no way to get from being sick to being well without feeling the feelings on their way out. If you're reading this book and thinking of how someone else could benefit from it, know that there's no rushing anyone into this process. It's a big commitment to be brave in the face of anxiety or depression. Someone must be sick enough to have the motivation to make the change. It is difficult to learn how to express feelings, to follow their path in the body and not panic. It was even hard for me to figure out what was a thought and what was a feeling at first. They were jumbled together and I had no idea when I was switching from one to the other.

Understanding the Normal Response to Trauma

The book, *Getting Unstuck: Unraveling the Knot of Depression, Attention and Trauma,* by Dr. Don Kerson was helpful. He explained that it was normal for people when traumatized or shamed to leave behind and separate from a part of oneself. In the end, most people will have many inner children inside that are abandoned and need to be reintegrated.

The fact that a psychiatrist was saying that this is a normal response to trauma, that there was a way out, and I could be helped was a game-changer. The biggest help was his exercise of visualizing the inner children I had left behind and reconnecting with them through a meditation process. We can visualize being in a safe place with these younger selves and comforting them. I practiced this regularly.

Constant Shaming for Being Human

As human beings, we all have fears, weaknesses and self-doubts. Unfortunately, in our society men are often shamed in their childhoods and beyond for expressing their fears or for crying. Both parents and peers can be belittling. Employers can too. Being shamed in childhood can lead to unconscious suppression of these feelings, so deeply that men might not be aware of it. They can dissociate—have the feelings go unconscious-- whenever uncomfortable feelings come up. Women face the same problems, for example, girls who are bold may face parental or teacher anger and peer shunning, again leading to unconscious suppression and dissociation. Depending on where or by whom we are raised, we can be shamed for being kind to people from different races, people who are overweight, or who have a disability. There's no end to whom it might not have been safe be kind to or identify with when we were children.

Suppressing Feelings Causes Inflammation

Suppressing feelings means whenever we have emotions, those messages that are not deemed acceptable are hidden from our awareness. This causes inflammation from accumulated neurochemicals that remain in the body until processed.

In more extreme cases of trauma, this could lead to domestic abuse or to hating people of the opposite sex because it wasn't safe to identify with a different gender, or people who have a physical or intellectual disability. As we head into an era where creativity is highly valued, we owe it to our boys and girls to teach them to accept a full range of emotional expression. It's best to develop our full capacity for tolerance, too. Without it we harm ourselves.

Our unconscious doesn't want to be punished, that's why it hides things from us. As soon as you create a safe space for your inner child, you'll be astonished at what starts to come up. Your body and mind want to process emotion and heal. All you have to do is learn how to safely get out of the way through processes like Dr. Kerson's visualizations, changing our negative self-talk, Focusing, John Barnes

MFR, and the rest of these mind-body tools I've been talking about.

Eye Movement Desensitization and Reprocessing (EMDR)

EMDR is a great tool for helping release trauma. It should be tried first with a psychotherapist, after which you can practice at home once you receive the go-ahead. The process is for the eyes to move side to side while you think of a difficult visual memory.

The normal way that adults store memories is to separate the visual memory of the event from the actual event. For people with PTSD, this separation doesn't occur. Recollection of the event recreates it, and our reaction, as if the event were happening all over again. Since it is quite common for anyone to have PTSD as the result of breaking a bone, divorce, or job loss, many of us could benefit from EMDR.

Francine Shapiro, the creator of EMDR says you can also move your eyes on the diagonal instead of just left and right, which I've found to be much more helpful than side-to-side.

How EMDR Can Help

As an example of how EMDR can potentially help you, here's how I used it to help me: at one traumatic point in my life, my PTSD was reactivated. I stopped being able to sleep through the REM cycle, where we do most of our dreaming. I woke up in a panic every night with a confusing jumble of disjointed anxiety-provoking images in my head. I stopped dreaming in color and instead had black and white images and static, like on an old TV. I couldn't tell my therapist about my dreams because the more I tried to retain the fragmented jumble, the more they evaporated. I found that if I focused on one image, I could retain it and think of it while I allowed myself to feel that panic. I paid attention to the feelings and whatever they did, however they changed and moved within me at the same time I did EMDR with diagonal eye movement. Diagonal eye movement worked much better for me that the typical left to right movement. I could feel a shift. I hoped that this would help me process what I needed to be working on so that I could start to sleep better. Sure enough, after a few months of doing it faithfully I started to have occasional flashes of color in my dreams and then over time, I started having regular dreams again, in color.

Focusing

Focusing is a form of healing therapy developed by Eugene Gendlin back in the 1970's. Focusing is learning how to attune to our emotions within our body, a formal practice of connecting with our body's own innate wisdom. It's looking for an internal awareness, a 'felt sense', asking ourselves how we are now, and welcoming however we are in the moment, no matter what feeling arises. According to Gendlin, a felt sense is a sense of unease or tension. It's something we distinctly feel, but is not clear to us. It's often unpleasant, strange or curious to begin with.

We can work by ourselves or with a friend but it is also possible to get training in how to focus and get paired with a partner through the Focusing Foundation. This is a relatively low-cost process for those with few resources who want good, solid results. There are also psychologists who combine therapy with Focusing for deep, lasting changes in our mental health and wellness. Focusing allows healing, and teaches us how to tune in to our internal guidance within a safe environment provided by a therapist, ourselves or a Focusing partner. Focusing helps us to connect with our creativity as well as making sure our body's emotional messages are received.

Sometimes we know how we feel. These are not times for Focusing. Those times are perfect for welcoming the feelings anyway, and allowing them to flow through us without judgment. When we have an unpleasant, strange or curious sensation, where we don't know how we feel, that is the perfect time to start Focusing. The body is receiving neurochemical emotional signals that it will ignore until we pay attention to our inner sense and sensations. Once we pay attention, the signals begin in earnest. We pause, and we stay with the experience. From this, we can learn to understand consciously what we really want at an unconscious level. It can help us integrate body, mind and spirit. Focusing can help us get more out of psychotherapy, and it can help us connect to our creativity. Tuning into all my emotions and body sensations non-judgmentally as Focusing teaches, has allowed me to get more out of many of the other therapies I've learned.

Life Coaches

While some people are enthusiastic about life coaches, at times I hear other people making fun of the people who use them. Many life coaches are therapists who have found that they don't like not being able to give good advice to people who are in pain and in great need of help. Building on strengths, as I discussed earlier, is a good way to go if you want to make serious changes in your life quickly. Being awakened to patterns of recurring self-sabotage so they can be healed is another way these coach/therapists can help.

Jungian Sandplay Therapy

My current therapist is a Jungian Analyst who uses Sandplay therapy in the style of Carl Jung and Dora Kalff. Sandplay therapy is a way of connecting to the unconscious when we feel stuck and unable to communicate with it via dreams. I have found the use of the sand trays, one filled with wet sand, the other with dry sand, combined with use of miniature figures and symbolic objects to be helpful to connect with my unconscious. The Jungian interpretation of dreams and view on the collective unconscious has also been an important part of what I needed to get well. Jungians encourage their clients to get body work, as it helps release and heal both mind and body, the conscious and unconscious. I sure wish I'd come across Jungian therapy sooner. Their deep connection to dreams and the collective unconscious is invaluable. For anyone interested in Jungian analysis, I'd suggest finding a therapist who incorporates dreams, active imagination, creative expression and sandplay therapy in the tradition of Carl Jung and Dora Kalff. I think it's a vital part of the connecting to the unconscious and the higher self.

One of the most important tools that I learned from my therapist was how to stay present in the body during stress. When something happens that cues a survival pattern, we can immediately check out of higher brain mode in a split second. Jungians call that survival pattern a complex. If we practice paying attention to our breath—not trying to change it, just noticing it, paying attention to gravity cues like the feeling of one's body in a chair or the sensations in our feet as we stand on the ground, we can stay in our higher brain. We might not always succeed at keeping out of the survival pattern, but the more we practice, the more capable we become. This is because we are growing new pathways in our brain as a result of a different response to the stimulus. Eventually we don't get triggered into our old behavior anymore.

Action Steps:
Easy:

Read *Getting Unstuck: Unraveling the Knot of Depression, Attention and Trauma,* by Dr. Don Kerson.

Read *Homecoming: Reclaiming and Healing Your Inner Child* by John Bradshaw.

Moderate:

Learn about Focusing. I'll suggest again reading *Focusing* by Eugene Gendlin or the book *How I Teach Focusing: Discovering the Gift of Your Inner Wisdom* by Bebe Simon.

Find a life coach and try a few sessions. I've enjoyed working with Kristina Coggins at klcoggins@mac.com. I've also been helped by Therese Skelly, who specializes in purpose-driven business coaching at happyinbusiness.com.

Harder:

Find a therapist you want to work with and start the process of healing. Try combining it with bodywork for the quickest results. Phone sessions allow you to completely connect to your body rather than be distracted by interacting with a therapist in person. I discovered Focusing through Dr. Ricki Morse, my partner's mother. Ricki is a PhD psychologist who has helped hundreds of people over the years using Focusing. She can be reached at rickpsyc@cox.net.

Find classes, other therapists, or a Focusing partner to work with through focusing.org.

Finding an analyst who also does sandplay is not easy. The IAAP—iaap.org--lists all certified analysts near you and you can interview them to make sure the body is a focus of theirs. Sandplay Therapists of America can be found at sandplay.org. The majority of sandplay therapists are not analysts, so be aware of that if it is important to you to work with an analyst. Analysts and therapists who've been trained in Marion Woodman's BodySoul process are another source of help. You can find them at mwoodmanfoundation.org.

Friday:

Improve Digestion and Nutrient Absorption

Chapter 21
Improving Digestion

I put the section of nutrition and digestion last because out of everything I've changed in my life, I've had the hardest time changing what I eat. I don't think that I am alone with this issue. We all need our comfort foods. For years I ate food that I knew was bad for me because I was emotionally starved and needed the comfort and feeling of acceptance and love that food gave me. I also ate because there were emotions I couldn't face and eating distracted me from facing them. I'm much better now than I was, but I still notice stress's effect on what, how much, and when I eat. I think it's a common human condition. As you read this section, remember to be encouraging to your inner child. It might feel overwhelming to look at the big picture I'm painting. Instead look for one small thing that resonates most if you feel you need digestive and nutritional changes. Making huge changes all at once seldom lasts. Taking small steps that build on each other over time is the way to create lasting change.

My Journey

I have had a huge struggle with digestion for most of my life. I used to lie on the cool marble floor of our house after supper when I was a little girl because it helped the stomachache I always got after eating. I thought that was normal. I remember going on dates when I was a teenager, eating the requisite pizza and soda and feeling like a bomb had gone off in my stomach. I thought that was normal too.

I had a bad bout of food poisoning in 2006. It is common for food poisoning to lead to a condition called SIBO, Small Intestinal Bacterial Overgrowth, due to the valve between the small intestine and large intestine being stuck open. This is one common cause of Irritable Bowel Syndrome (IBS.) I suffered from IBS attacks for a year, making several trips to the emergency room, before it was diagnosed by a gastroenterologist. Now that you have my history as a digestive tract sufferer, you know why I have spent a lot of time researching how to get better.

Why Timing of Water is Critical

Even if your digestion works well, you can make it better. Drink 12 ounces of water 15 to 30 minutes before eating. This is a tip I learned from my Ayurvedic doctor, Dr. John Douillard, who told me that the stomach has a layer of tissue that acts as a pool of bicarbonate, a protective layer that insures that stomach acid cannot burn a hole through the stomach.

Our brain has a biofeedback mechanism to tell if this tissue is properly hydrated or not. It needs to be fully hydrated to be protective. If it is not fully hydrated, the brain will dial down the stomach acid strength.

Stomach Acid to Bile Connection

We need stomach acid at full strength to break down the food into absorbable nutrients. Good quality bile is only possible with full strength stomach acid. Over time, if we have not done a good job about being hydrated we do not have the bile quality needed. Bile and stomach acids are necessary so we can digest and absorb building blocks for our body. Years of going without full strength stomach acid (either because we are poor water drinkers or because of taking too many antacids or acid blockers due to heartburn or acid reflux), means we have been harming our health. We have nowhere near the stockpile of nutrients we need to stay healthy and keep any genetic disposition we have toward illness at bay.

Other Problems Caused by Not Drinking Enough Water

When we do not drink enough water it also causes our bile to get thicker, which can lead to gallstones clogging up our gall bladder. Whenever we eat, bile gets released into the food that is about to enter our small intestine. The fattier the food is, the more bile gets released. Bile is alkaline and is meant to neutralize the acidity of the food/stomach acid mixture. It cannot do its job if it is too thick or if our gallbladder is clogged with gallstones.

For years I had low cholesterol, a combined HDL and LDL of 137. Cholesterol is needed by the body for proper function. Cholesterol is important for keeping skin healthy. I used to get horribly deep cracks in my skin particularly in winter because of inadequate cholesterol, but that's changed since working with Dr. Douillard because my cholesterol levels have normalized. We need cholesterol to produce hormones such as adrenaline, testosterone and estrogen too, so if our cholesterol levels are too low, we may have low hormone levels.

I believe that our brain sends hunger signals until it senses it has the nutrients it needs. If the brain does not get what it needs, it is going to keep sending signals to eat. I certainly notice that when I eat nutrient-dense foods, I'm satisfied sooner. Also, if we do not chew our food thoroughly, our body can't digest it enough to provide us the nutrients we need. I try my best to chew thoroughly. I try to wait until I'm hungry to eat, but not too hungry, because then I'm in a hurry and eat too quickly. In rebuilding my health, I've found that when I eat pureed vegetable soups that I do not eat as big a meal as I do when I skip soups or don't puree them. The nutrients in pureed foods are more easily absorbed compared to hastily or incompletely chewed food.

The Negative Impact of Poor Digestion on the Immune System

Something else I learned from Dr. Douillard is that if we do not produce enough bile to neutralize stomach acid or if the bile is too thick, or there are too many gallstones, the food entering our small intestine will be too acidic. When this happens, the small intestine will produce mucus to protect itself.

The problem with having mucus in our small intestine is that 80% of our immune system is in the first part of our small intestine. It's in tissue called GALT (Gut Associated Lymphatic Tissue). GALT is the central command zone for our lymphatic system. GALT is supposed to pull off any toxins in our food. If it is covered with mucus however, there is no way that any toxins are being pulled off.

This means that if we have these kinds of digestive issues: making insufficient bile, a clogged gallbladder, or thickened bile, we are digesting toxins. It makes sense that anyone who suffers from bad digestion should start eating organic food to reduce their intake of toxins, if they are not already doing so.

You may feel abdominal discomfort after a fatty meal - this is often in the liver and gallbladder regions as the gallbladder struggles to release bile, but can't because the ducts are clogged with thick bile or gallstones.

It is hard to get back to feeling good once your gallbladder is clogged or you have poor quality bile. An intestinal cleanse and gall bladder flush are helpful to relieve this. I do this yearly through Dr. Douillard's online program, although some people do this twice a year. Contact info is in the action steps at the end of this chapter.

The Impact of Chronic Stress on Digestion

Again, chronic stress means we are in a state of fight or flight or freeze. Under chronic stress, our brain is primed to use the primitive and emotional parts of the dominant hemisphere of our brain, so we're not thinking as clearly and rationally as we could be. Our primitive brain and emotional brain were not meant to be used so constantly, which starts an inflammatory response within the brain.

Adrenals Win Out Over Digestion

Digestion is halted when we are in fight or flight. In this state, blood is sent to the legs and arms so we can escape from a predator instead of to our digestive tract. The blood moves away from the digestive tract. Adrenaline needs to be made from cholesterol and that takes a lot of vitamin C to make. As a result, the digestive tract becomes undersupplied with vitamin C as well as B vitamins. If we were really running away from a predator our bodies would burn off the adrenaline, but since our boss and coworkers are not officially predators, the cholesterol that is used to make adrenaline gets coated onto our arteries. (If we had healthy amounts of lecithin in our bodies, the cholesterol could pass on through our arterial walls, so our body could make use of it, but we need adequate amounts of choline and inosotol, two B vitamins, to make lecithin.) Many of us have a genetic need for high amounts of some B vitamins, or a reduced ability to process B vitamins to their usable methylated state.

The Downward Spiral

Without the blood on hand we need to digest food, without the nutrients for a healthy digestive tract, with fascial tension so high that cells can't properly operate, we start a downward spiral in the health of our digestive tract.

The tissue is less healthy because it is not getting enough blood, vitamin C or B vitamins. If it is not healthy it cannot absorb nutrients as well as it should. If it is not getting enough water to stay optimally hydrated, food gets stuck in the digestive tract and does not move as fast as it should. That means bacteria can proliferate and attack the walls of the small and large intestines.

Pockets of infection can start up. Because of being on high alert and pumped up on adrenaline, our bodies never get the signal that it is time for a repair cycle. We need to be in a parasympathetic nervous system state (PNS) to not only digest but to repair our small and large intestines to remove and repair damaged cilia. Being in sympathetic nervous system (SNS) dominance means staying in an inflammatory, constantly degrading physical state. This can lead to leaky gut syndrome.

Excess use of NSAIDs (non-steroidal anti-inflammatories

such as aspirin or ibuprofen) can cause leaky gut due to the spaces between the digestive tissue widening. Excessive use of antibiotics can cause both non-beneficial bacteria and yeast to thrive; it can also cause leaky gut. Lectins (a low-grade toxin used by plants to protect themselves from over-foraging) found in most plants can cause leaky gut and interfere with nutrient absorption. Lectins are also found in animals to help support immunological functions and assist in protein synthesis and delivery. Small amounts of lectins in the foods we eat are fine; it's when there are large quantities that they can prevent us from absorbing nutrients in our food. Traditionally, the most problematic foods were soaked or fermented to help inactivate the lectins. Lectins are most concentrated in foods like beans, (especially soy), grains (especially wheat), nuts, dairy, and the nightshade family (eggplant, tomatoes, potatoes, peppers, tomatillos) and GMO foods, where lectins can be spliced in to protect food from pests. Some people have found relief from autoimmune illness by avoiding high lectin foods, according to Joseph Cohen in *The Self-Hacked Secrets*.

Diets that are high in hard-to-digest foods like dairy or wheat can also tax the digestive tract if we are under chronic stress.

Peristalsis

Our digestive tract is quite athletic when we are healthy. The motion of the digestive tract is called peristalsis and the muscles used in peristalsis are stimulated by insoluble fiber. Over time, the lack of regularly eating high-fiber green leafy vegetables can catch up with us and our digestive tract can get flabby and out of shape.

If the digestive tract is struggling to recover from food poisoning or long-term neglect, sudden intake of large quantities of insoluble fiber like popcorn can set off a stomachache if not an outright IBS attack. If our digestive muscles are kept in good shape by regularly eating insoluble fiber, particularly leafy greens, and regularly taking probiotics, then these kinds of problems are unlikely to crop up.

Chronic Stress, Muscle Tension and Fascial Tension

Muscle tension in the body can also impact digestion. In particular, fight-or-flight muscles like the psoas can cause tension through the abdomen and restrict proper movement of food through the digestive tract. Fascia can also bind the muscles around the digestive tract and keep them from moving properly. I think of this as another benefit of RFST, yoga, and meditation: improved digestion when fascial and muscle tension decrease. Fascial tension impacts us down to the cellular level, because there is fascia around each cell.

Muscle tension can also be caused by too little magnesium. Again, this can happen over time from our digestion going wrong because of being in a sympathetic nervous system dominant state. This kind of muscle tension, together with the fascial tension that chronic stress causes, can be a driver of reduced blood flow and therefore reduced oxygenation for muscles, tendons, ligaments, joints and bone. I believe it can lead to degenerative conditions like arthritis as well as playing a part in autoimmune disorders.

The Importance of Healthy Bacteria in our GI Tract

There is a need to make sure that the digestive bacteria (called the microbiome) that we inherited is kept healthy and vibrant. More and more though, after multiple generations of antibiotic use in humans and livestock, the quality of the microbiome we inherit is not so great. It has been shown that good bacteria tend to die off when we are stressed. Freeloading bad bacteria are more vigorous, so they step in and take over.

It is important to reduce our stress load and identify if we experience intestinal gas and bloating. If we notice an increase in the quantity of intestinal gas, there are steps we can take to identify the culprits and get rid of them because they are starving us of vital nutrients. Taking over-the-counter medications and ignoring the general trend of our digestion leads to chronic ill health. I think we are at the mercy of our genetic weaknesses when we do not provide our bodies with the building blocks to stay healthy. It sends us down the pipeline into inflammation and ill health.

UCLA researchers have found that gut bacteria alter people's brain function. Other research has found that a type of bacteria called Lactobacillus rhamnosus positively impacts GABA levels and lowers the stress-induced hormone corticosterone, which in turn reduced anxiety and depression-related behavior in test subjects. Some psychologists now treat anxiety and depression in part with probiotic therapy.

It's more widely known that psychologists have encouraged their clients to use meditation, journaling, and high intensity aerobic exercise. Perhaps part of the benefit these activities provide is that reducing stress helps the good gut bacteria to thrive again. According to Dr. Maggie Phillips, a psychologist who specializes in trauma recovery, psychologists have found that combining probiotic use and psychotherapy together has reduced symptoms of depression enough to require no traditional psychotherapeutic drugs within six months, with psychotherapy/probiotic treatment concluded after one year.

Histamine Intolerance

Histamine is a compound that our body makes. It acts as a neurotransmitter, regulates function in the gut, and plays a vital part of our local immune alert response. Histamine also occurs naturally in food, even very healthy foods. Our ability to handle histamines in our food is reduced when we are stressed.

Since histamine is a part of the trigger that activates our sympathetic nervous system, eating foods high in histamine can put us on the pathway toward inflammation, poor nutritional absorption, anemia, low iron, low calcium, low magnesium, low B-12, leaky gut and osteoporosis. This happens particularly when we are chronically stressed. Excess histamine in our diet beyond what we can process causes inflammation and damage in our intestinal tract. It plays a big part of reducing our body's ability to repair itself.

A damaged intestinal tract cannot digest food as well as a healthy, uninflamed one can. Our western diet is rich in histamines which occur naturally in aged foods like vinegar and cheese, smoked meats, cultured foods like yogurt, kefir and buttermilk, pickled foods and fermented foods like wine, beer, kombucha, and soy sauce. They are also found in citrus fruits as well as avocado, tomatoes, strawberries, raspberries, cherries and apricots.

As foods age, they become higher in histamines, so it's important for people with histamine intolerance to buy fresh foods, cook what is needed and try not to eat leftovers. We can freeze leftovers if necessary because freezing cooked foods halts histamine formation, but we need to eat these foods within a month. Lots of meats are aged to become more tender, so we need to use caution and ask questions of our butcher when buying meat. Buying fresh meat, or meat aged no more than 1-2 weeks after being butchered can make a difference, as can buying fish no more than 12 hours old.

The Importance of DAO and HNMT

Diamine oxidase (DAO) and histamine N-methyltransferase are enzymes that the body makes to break down histamine. It is common to take medications that block our ability to break down histamines, like NSAIDs (aspirin, ibuprofen/Advil, Aleve) and other medications like cimetidine, dihydralazine, NKC heparin and some chemotherapy drugs. It might be a good idea for cancer patients to ask their doctor and nutritionist if they should watch for excess dietary histamines and to build DAO as much as possible.

It is also important to make sure to get enough vitamin C, B-6, zinc, copper and magnesium in our diets to support production of DAO. DAO is made in the small intestine by the body, but if the small intestine is damaged from chronic stress or mucus buildup because of bile not doing its job, then DAO production will not be optimized. DAO-supporting foods are olive oil and pea shoots grown without light.

It might be that one of the Mediterranean diet's biggest benefits comes from the protective quality of olive oil in maximizing DAO production and keeping the intestinal tract healthy.

HNMT is an enzyme concentrated in the liver and is responsible for breaking down histamine in the nervous system. It's possible to have too little of it too. Things like DAO deficiency, bacterial imbalances, HNMT genetic inheritance and HNMT inhibitors like the drugs diphenhydramine (found in Benadryl), amodiaquine (an antimalarial), and tacrine (an early Alzheimer's drug), can all reduce the amount of HNMT in the body.

Some people get obvious symptoms of histamine intolerance, like flushing after drinking some types of red wine that are high in sulfates, or they get hives when exposed to histamines, but many people don't have anything so obvious happen. If you suspect you might have a problem with histamine, you might be impacted the way I was. I didn't have flushing or hives, but I was frequently sick. I never connected that my coughing or having a slightly runny nose after eating had any meaning other than I was getting another cold. I had no idea why some foods made me produce phlegm. Since learning about the problem and making the connection, I can see that my histamine reaction was leading me to get sick. Many times, I've had a histamine intolerance reaction from the first bite of balsamic vinaigrette on a lettuce leaf. I start coughing uncontrollably and wheezing. Despite drinking water to try to flush away the irritating balsamic, it directly leads to a week-long sore throat and sinus infection. For me, the balsamic vinegar hits the back of my throat, my body starts to attack it like it's an invader, my throat swells up with inflammation and the area becomes easy pickings for whatever bacteria is on site to penetrate the tissue. My immune system is already overwhelmed by constant invasion due to leaky gut, so in overreacting to the balsamic it misses the offending bacteria and voila, yet another cold.

Extra Virgin Olive Oil

I've added in several tablespoons a day of cold pressed extra virgin olive oil, usually to my salad, as a way of upping my DAO production. I find it helpful in reducing my symptoms both digestively and improving my quality of sleep (side effects of high histamine levels include anxiety and insomnia.) I'm adding organic pea sprouts, too, although it is incredibly inconvenient to grow them, so it's not as frequently as I'd like. Make sure to buy the kind of pea seeds meant for sprouting so they're not chemically treated. And if you find you have trouble with acid reflux, which can be connected to high histamine levels, ask your doctor if you should try melatonin. Studies show that taking melatonin is just as effective toward reducing acid reflux or heartburn as medication like Prevacid, and it might help your sleep.

Action Steps:
Easy:
   If your doctor approves, add 1-2 tablespoons of olive oil and a probiotic to your daily diet. Chew your food well. Consider melatonin for your heartburn.
   Time your water intake to help rebuild your stomach acid and bile production.
   Read *Spark* by John Ratey, MD. Dr. Ratey advocates high-intensity aerobic exercise for a number of conditions.
   Read *The Self-Hacked Secrets*, by Joseph Cohen.
   Read Mark Sissman's excellent blog at MarksDailyApple.com for more information about lectins and other nutritional advice with a paleo perspective.

Medium:
   If you have insomnia or anxiety, consider timing when you eat higher histamine foods so that you're consuming them in the morning and at lunchtime rather than loading up on them at night. The caveat here is that I believe the worst part of my leaky gut is located in a particular section of my digestive tract. It takes about 6-7 hours of digestion time to reach it, just perfect for me to wake up at 3 a.m. to anxiety and insomnia.
   If you have leaky gut and you've tried making other changes

without success, try figuring out if you've got a similar situation. This is part of the reason that eating dinner like a pauper as Dr. Douillard recommends (ideally for me a small, simple dinner low in histamines which includes pea sprouts and olive oil) helps me get a better night's sleep. Try an intestinal cleanse and gallbladder flush. There are lots of Ayurvedic doctors in the US. You can look them up online by using the search terms "Ayurvedic doctors in the USA." Dr. Douillard's program is available through his website, lifespa.com.

Harder:

Stop eating leftovers if you have a problem with histamine.

We need the nutrition found in histamine-rich foods in order to heal, but it makes sense to reduce intake of high histamine foods which are not particularly nutritious, like beer and wine, until you heal.

Stop using aged foods like balsamic vinegar and switch to fresh cheese when possible instead of aged cheese. You can get information on the latest research, great advice on how to heal, as well as nutritious recipes that appeal to both men and women at healinghistamine.com, run by Yasmina Ykelenstam, a former news journalist who became a health journalist after her own histamine issues forced her to research her way back to health.

Mindbodygreen.com also has some excellent resources about histamine and DAO.

Dr. Maggie Phillips is at maggiephillipsphd.com.

Chapter 22
Nutrition You Can Live With

Our Unique Bodies

It's become clear to me that we are all so unique that there's no one diet right for everyone. The combination of genes and gut flora we inherited can make what heals one person hurt someone else. I've had to learn how to listen to my body, and it's hard to do because I've found that often what we eat doesn't impact us for days, or weeks, or even months. What is true for everyone is that we can improve our body's ability to digest food and provide balanced blood sugar by getting out of constant sympathetic nervous system activation. No matter what type of diet we follow, it's clear that no one thrives on sugar and processed foods. I've cut back on these to a bare minimum. Instead, I look to eat plenty of nutrient-dense foods every day to provide my body the best chance it has at getting the building blocks it needs to maintain my health.

Look for the ANDI food score, which rates foods for nutritional density. It's available at drfuhrman.com. If you suspect you have leaky gut, you might need to be vigilant about what types of food you choose from the ANDI scale. For example, kale has the highest nutritional density, but if you choose curly kale, it is high in oxalates, which I am sensitive to. Lacinato/dinosaur kale is the type I use, though I don't use it much raw because it's not great for the thyroid. More explanation on oxalates is in the next chapter.

Stabilizing Blood Sugar

It is important to stabilize our blood sugar for the health of our body and brain. This means limiting our sugar and refined carbohydrate intake. High sugar intake has been linked to heart disease, though for years the blame was put on fat. Blood sugar swings from eating sugar and refined carbohydrates have also been shown to damage the brain. For people who have blood sugar swings or who are light sleepers, the Ayurvedic suggestion to eat breakfast like a prince, lunch like a king, and dinner like a pauper might be of help. When I first tried this, it helped me sleep better because it helped stabilize my blood sugar levels as well as lessening the discomfort of digesting a large meal at night, which can disturb light sleepers. I believe that people with autoimmune diseases are most likely to be sympathetic nervous system dominant, which means they will have more of an issue with blood sugar stabilization. I've found that to be true for me, so I'm careful about avoiding most simple carbohydrates. I try to make sure the carbs I eat count, for example, by including resistant starch (a type of starch we can't digest which stays in our gut longer) in the mix to help feed good gut bacteria.

Getting Individualized Help on What to Eat

Over time, we might develop food hypersensitivities that keep our digestive tracts irritated and unable to repair themselves. These sensitivities are unique to each of us. If you are already sick, it could be of benefit to find out which foods are helpful and which foods are inflammatory for you. I got a lot of help from Dr. James Roach of Midway, Kentucky, better known as America's Doctor, on what not to eat so my body could heal. He gave me a blood test called the IgE to find out if I had hypersensitivities. When he discussed the results with me, it was clear that I did. It helped to know exactly what I could safely eat. The results were given as a list of common foods categorized into high, medium and low inflammatory response. Some examples from my testing: no type of milk was okay. I'd thought goats' milk yogurt was fine, but the tests show that I had a high level of response to it. I had high reactivity to cherries, lots of types of beans as well as some herbs like rosemary that I was unaware of. I've made some big changes because of these findings. It wasn't hard to give up things like cherries, beans and rosemary because I'm not overly fond of any of them. I needed good proof to give up yogurt because it was my go-to food. After I gave up eating those inflammatory foods, I felt noticeably better. I still have yogurt as a treat every few months, but it's less appealing to me because I've seen how much better I feel without it. I'd tried giving up yogurt before, but couldn't see a difference in how I felt, because I was still eating so many other things that irritated my body. The tests Dr. Roach ordered also showed what nutrients I was deficient in. Among other things, I was surprised to learn I had very low copper levels. Dr. Roach gave me directions on which supplements to take to help rebuild my health. More information about Dr. Roach is in action steps of this chapter.

Vegan Diets, Insoluble and Soluble Fiber

Some people are helped by vegan diets, but I had IBS attacks when I tried it because my body couldn't handle the insoluble fiber. I have a friend who's got a new lease on life thanks to his vegan diet, though. It's greatly improved his blood chemistry after discovering he had a clogged "widowmaker" left anterior descending artery.

When my life is in good balance, I can handle more raw vegetables in my diet. When I'm stressed, I can't. When I make a mistake in what I eat, I've been lucky to identify a soluble fiber (acacia fiber) that doesn't upset my stomach. Plenty of people can't use it, though, because they may have freeloading gut flora that like to eat acacia fiber. If you have trouble digesting foods with insoluble fiber, try hunting for a soluble fiber that helps you. Make sure to have some whenever you eat insoluble fiber. Some people swear by konjac flour, also called glucomannan. Whatever you buy, look for a reputable source. A good intro book to explain insoluble fiber and soluble fiber is *Help for IBS*, by Heather Van Vorous. I take some of the book's information with a grain of salt, because she promotes wheat as being soothing during an IBS attack, while I know that wheat makes me feel worse during an IBS attack, plus leads to sinus infections for me. She only suggests acacia fiber as a soluble fiber, but I know that some people can't use it, though for me it's been a godsend. Those issues aside, her book does a very good job of differentiating between foods with soluble and insoluble fiber, which foods are trigger foods, and how to calm the gut. As an example, her book helped me find my go-to foods when I was in the middle of an IBS attack: applesauce and instant oatmeal with no added sugar. As suggested in *Help for IBS,* I've also found that small meals were essential when I had an ongoing attack, and I frequently sipped water with acacia fiber added, so that I rarely had a totally empty digestive tract. If you suspect you might have IBS, Heather's book is a great place to start educating yourself. I also found her peppermint capsules (taken with food) and her fennel seed tea to be a big help during an IBS attack or to stave off an IBS attack.

Diets

I've been asked what my favorite diet is. I'd love to say the Mediterranean diet, but as much as I love its health benefits, I think that as they age, for people who have been traumatized, the Mediterranean diet is a prescription for weight gain. Many of us can no longer eat wheat, and gluten-free replacements, while much more palatable than they used to be, are often even more likely than wheat to cause weight gain. We also need to be careful with portion sizes on fruits, even low sugar ones like apples, berries, watermelon and cantaloupe.

I believe there's hope--that it's not so much that people's metabolisms always get slow as they age, but instead, it's that we're seeing that accumulated traumas cause the vagus nerve to be suppressed, which means blood sugar is no longer balanced. Trauma might also reduce the tendency to exercise, given that traumatized people are more likely to have chronic health issues that might discourage or prevent them from exercising. Research has shown that muscle mass doesn't have to take a downturn until about the age of seventy. That's a sign that we have more capacity than we think to keep our metabolism elevated. If we can put the long-term effort into healing, I believe we can reactivate our vagal tone, and along with a balanced exercise program and a healthy microbiome, reawaken our metabolic rate back to a normal level.

Pro-Veg, Pro-Organic

You could call what I eat a modified Mediterranean-Paleo diet. In general, I aim for a diet with lots of vegetables, some organic chicken, wild fish, and grass-fed meat. 100% grass fed beef is full of omega 3 fatty acids rather than the omega 6 fatty acids found in grain-fed beef. Our diets are too high in omega 6 fatty acids, so it's nice to have another source for omega 3's. I do not fear fat in a phobic way like a lot of people do these days, but neither am I eating lots of fat and meat at every meal. I'm careful of the fats I eat because I still don't make enough bile. I take milk thistle whole-herb capsules to try to improve my bile production. I've made sure to get olive oil in my daily diet, along with some coconut oil, which is full of medium chain fatty acids that are good for the brain. I add bioflavonoids as suggested by the research findings Yasmina Ykelenstam reports about on her website Healing Histamine. You could say I'm cautiously paleo, trying for 60% vegetables in my diet. I need to limit the carbs in my diet because of problems with hypoglycemia and a genetic tendency towards type 2 diabetes. My hypoglycemia is almost non-existent since I started intermittent fasting, eating only in an eight-hour window between noon and 8pm. I start off the morning with what I think of as an improvement on the Bulletproof coffee recipe and then aim for lunch at noon. Intermittent fasting has been shown to help people with diabetes, heart disease, epilepsy, fatty liver disease, and helps inhibit growth and spread of a type of childhood leukemia called acute lymphoblastic leukemia.

It is important to find balance however you eat. It seems that the biggest problem with red meat is that it encourages the growth of a type of digestive bacteria that raises our triglyceride levels; at least the grain-fed version does. The more red meat we eat, the higher those levels of bacteria and therefore the higher our triglyceride levels, which are inflammatory to our body.

Impact of our Intestinal Biome on our Mood and Cravings

It is important to realize the significance of bacteria in our bodies and how they interact with our DNA. Yeast overgrowth is more likely each time we use antibiotics if we do not continuously reseed with probiotics while we take the antibiotics. Yeast overgrowth is also more likely to occur because of high fructose corn syrup intake and high amounts of other sugars in our typical Western diet.

The bacteria and yeast in our bodies can affect the size of our appetite. Some bacteria and yeast are beneficial, but others are freeloaders and create poisonous toxins. One type of bacteria, C. dificile, is associated with a muscle stiffness found with autistic spectrum kids. The only way to have the good kind of bacteria is to feed it what it likes, (sadly, not sugar and processed foods) and the only way to get rid of the bad kind is to starve it by not eating what it likes (which means no or low sugar and processed foods.) Colonic irrigation and reseeding with probiotics can help that process along.

The good kind of gut bacteria is much more susceptible to dying off with stress than the bad kind--and that includes internal stress. This is another reason why it is critical to nurture our inner child and be careful about how we speak to ourselves. Reducing internal stress around eating can help improve the quality of our diet (for example, I respond better to self-encouragement to eat better next time when I make a poor food choice rather than shaming myself for having made a mistake.) Reducing internal stress helps me have a healthier microbiome. As everyone knows, it's best to stay away from the processed food aisles.

Rethink Dairy and Wheat

It's a good idea to rethink dairy and wheat at least until we regain our health, because both are inflammatory. Dairy can cause a cycle of constipation if our bile is poor quality or too thick. Without the right amount of good quality bile, fat will not be fully absorbed by the small intestine. This makes the body shut down peristalsis until all the fat is absorbed. Since fat is a liquid in the body, the body also absorbs additional water from our stool, leading to constipation.

Both wheat and dairy can cause immune issues if we have leaky gut syndrome. The particles can get into the body and cause a release of histamine, which creates mucus and congestion in our sinuses, leading to sinus infections. An example from my life: it took me three and a half months without wheat to notice a difference in my sinus health. But once I did, I have not had to take antibiotics for a sinus infection since, and that was seven years ago.

In my experience, as I've released more abdominal fascia, I've realized that fascial tension can keep us from proper peristalsis, which could contribute to problems with constipation or diarrhea. The more abdominal fascia I've released, particularly around the psoas muscles, the healthier my digestion has become.

The Benefits of Unrefined Salt and Iodine

In the book, *Salt Your Way to Health,* Dr. David Brownstein says, "Refined salt leads to nutritional deficiencies in trace minerals as well as sodium imbalance in your body"

Many commercial bread products are made using bromide which confuses the body. Our body needs iodine, but bromide and iodine are similar enough that the body will use bromide instead of iodine, especially if iodine is undersupplied, as it tends to be in the western world. The thyroid needs iodine. Bromide inhibits the thyroid; the thyroid is responsible for our metabolism, so if we eat commercial bread products we may be reducing the activity of our thyroid.

This means we are lowering our metabolism, which could cause us to gain weight. Some states, like California, have banned the use of bromides or bromates in bread. In other states, buyer beware. It might be a good reason to bake your own bread using bromide-free flour. Ask your Ayurvedic doctor if he recommends supplementing with iodine—I've only found Ayurvedic doctors to be versed enough in its use to recommend it at high levels. Never take extra iodine beyond what's in table salt without talking to an Ayurvedic doctor first, because it's toxic if unneeded.

Dr. Brownstein recommends Celtic Sea Salt from Selina Naturally or Real Salt by Redmond Trading Company. Using regular iodized salt and adding in trace minerals like ancient sea minerals from your local health food store is a good compromise.

Iodine and Breast Cancer Rates

Japanese women have four to five times lower rates of breast cancer than women in the United States. They get a lot more iodine in their diet than U.S. women because of their seaweed consumption. Ayurvedic doctors think that feeding iodine to the thyroid reduces fibrocystic breast disease which reduces breast cancer risk. I had fibrocystic breast disease until I started taking iodine at Dr. Douillard's recommendation.

My gynecologist requested an ultrasound as well as a mammogram the first year that ultrasounds were offered because my breast tissue had always been dense and filled with cystic tissue. This was ten months after I had started taking iodine. When the ultrasound results came in they told me my breast tissue was normal and that I did not need to have an ultrasound again. In the years since I have never been asked to have another ultrasound.

Medical Herbology

We can be aided in our quest to heal by learning which medical herbs (no, I'm not referring to marijuana) can assist our conditions. Herbs such as ginger can help with digestion. Slippery elm bark and herbal licorice can soothe the tissue of our digestive tract. Hawthorne is helpful for the heart. There are wonderful herbologists out there who are teaching people what they can do for themselves through identifying local plants and creating their own tinctures and salves. Medical herbologists can also advise which herbs are right for their clients and where they can find reputable sources to buy. I had the privilege of taking classes from Janice Ditchek when I lived in New York. She works with a local doctor too, to assist his patients. I really enjoyed her classes.

Action Steps:
Easy:

Enjoy seaweed salads regularly and change to sea salt if your doctor approves, making sure to replace the iodine with seaweed or a supplement.

Be good about taking a daily probiotic. Add bioflavonoids to your diet. Ask your doctor if you should switch to bread made without bromide.

Moderate:

If you have blood sugar issues, try a consultation with an Ayurvedic doctor.

Try John Barnes MFR if you think you might have fascial restrictions in your abdomen. More at myofascialrelease.com.

Read the blog at marksdailyapple.com for sensible ways to reduce over-reliance on processed carbs—handy even if you're not paleo.

I've found Dr. Josh Axe's website to be helpful for nutritional information. You can find him at draxe.com.

See an integrative medicine specialist for potential IgG food hypersensitivities. Dr. Jim Roach can be contacted at themidwaycenter.com.

If you think you might have IBS, read *Help for IBS* and talk to your doctor. It can take a long time to get diagnosed. Patient awareness can help point your doctor in the right direction and reduce the time it takes to get a diagnosis.

Contact Janice Ditchek for a session or to sign up for a class at jditchek@gmail.com.

Harder:

Try rethinking your diet if you have signs of leaky gut syndrome. Ask your doctor if it's okay for you to add chlorophyll and/or chamomile tea to your diet. Both help the body repair the squamous epithelial cells that line our GI tract. I use the broken cell wall type of chlorophyll so it's easier for my body to get nutrition from it. A word of caution: I have to take soluble fiber with my chlorophyll. For me, chlorophyll powder alone feels like each particle comes with its own tiny chainsaw. Most people have no problems with chamomile tea, but it started causing tachycardia for me, so I had to stop using it.

Add a good protein powder to your daily diet. I'll be posting the recipe for the one I make for my smoothie on my book's website yourbesthealthbyfriday.com.

Sign up to attend Dr. Roach's health seminar. The information is accessible to laypeople even though most of the attendees are doctors and naturopaths looking to gain the knowledge needed to prevent disease rather than trying to fix problems after the fact. More info at themidwaycenter.com.

Chapter 23
Internal Repair

Help for Irritable Bowel Syndrome (IBS) Woes

For those who have IBS, it's common at unexpected times to have large quantities of gas. Social situations can be a nightmare because sufferers never know when it is going to strike or which foods are going to cause a problem. Among other reasons, odor could be a sign of inadequate stores of vitamins for the liver to produce albumen. (Albumen is needed to remove waste through urination.) It might be a sign that we aren't eating enough protein to allow for efficient peristalsis, (normal contraction of the digestive tract) to move food along. If that's the case, the food stays in the intestine long enough that some amount of decay sets in. It's also possible that past antibiotic use has allowed the digestive tract to be colonized by bad bacteria, or we're not drinking enough water, or some combination of all the above.

Seek the Help of Integrative Medicine Doctors, Fusion Medicine Doctors, Ayurvedic doctors and Naturopaths

Integrative medicine doctors, Ayurvedic doctors, fusion or functional medicine doctors and naturopaths can help us work on nutritional needs and rebuilding digestive capacity. Trying the BED (Body Ecology Diet) or GAPS (Gut and Psychology Syndrome) diet can help too. Elimination diets like the BED or GAPS diet are not easy, so it's important to be extra kind and patient with ourselves.

It's not uncommon to have a sense of fear or failure when

trying something new like an elimination diet, even while under a doctor's guidance, so our inner critics may be very active. Heaping on self-praise and keeping a gratitude journal with at least three things you are grateful for every day can be a help in anything new you try. If you try an elimination diet, you might encourage yourself by telling yourself that each day you follow it is one step closer to figuring out your path to better health.

Why we Should Care about Glycoproteins

Glycoproteins are sugar molecules attached to protein molecules. They are essential for your body to properly function. Here are a few examples of what glycoproteins do: they're vital for white blood cell recognition, our antibodies are glycoproteins, they help bind fibers and cells of connective tissues and help calcium in connective tissue bind to bone. Many of our hormones are glycoproteins and they are an important component of mucus produced throughout the body.

From what I've read, it appears the body does best if it is stocked with the essential ingredients to make its own glycoproteins (which includes eight essential sugars, also called glycans, such as xylose, fucose, galactose, glucose, mannose, n-acetylglucosamine, n-acetylgalactosamine and n-acetylneuraminic acid.)

Xylose is found in guava, pears, blackberries, loganberries, raspberries, aloe vera, echinacea, boswellia, psyllium seeds, broccoli, spinach, eggplant, peas, green beans, okra, cabbage and corn. It's said to prevent cancer of the digestive system.

Fucose is found in brown seaweed like kelp and wakame, some mushrooms and seeds. It helps support long-term memory and fights allergies.

Galactose is found in plums, mango, orange, prunes, peach, rhubarb, cranberries, blackberries, raspberries, apples, currants, dates, pineapple, kiwi, apricot, pear, strawberries, passionfruit, Echinacea, chestnuts, leaks, onions, brussels sprouts, green beans, carrots, eggplant, cauliflower, asparagus, broccoli, avocado, celery, cucumber,

196

potato, tomatoes, beets, mushrooms, parsnips and green peas. It's said to improve the speed of healing from injuries as well as improve memory.

Mannose is found in blackcurrants, red currants, gooseberries and cranberries, aloe vera, green beans, cabbage, eggplant, tomatoes and turnips. It helps reduce inflammation and reduces disease through its anti-bacterial, anti-fungal and anti-viral properties.

Glucose is found in honey, grapes, banana, mangoes, cherries, strawberries, cocoa, aloe vera, licorice, sasparilla, hawthorn, garlic and Echinacea. Glucose is best eaten as part of a whole food rather than as table sugar stripped of fiber and nutrients.

N-acetylneuraminic acid is found in whey protein isolate and chicken eggs, as well as human breast milk. It's anti-bacterial and anti-viral and is said to be important in brain function, particularly brain development and learning.

N-acetyl-galactosamine is found in shark cartilage and bovine cartilage. Either one can be problematic to find a good, safe source, so be cautious if you're thinking of supplementing this. N-acetyl-galactosamine is reported to inhibit the spread of tumors, regulate inflammation and help immune system functioning.

N-acetyl-glucosamine is found in shitake mushrooms and glucosamine sulfate. It's said to help the immune system, repair cartilage and the mucosal lining damaged by ulcerative colitis and Crohn's Disease.

Unfortunately, modern wheat contains inflammatory glycoproteins whether it is white or whole wheat according to Dr. Mark Hyman. Eating sugar and other high processed foods also increases the amount of inflammatory proteins that circulate in our bodies.

Just as we need a proper balance of omega-3, 6 and 9 fatty acids in our diet, we need a proper balance of healthy glycoproteins and glycans (those essential sugars I mentioned earlier.) Unfortunately, in the same way our Western diets are weighted too heavily towards omega-6 fatty acids, which causes inflammation, our diets are weighted much too heavily towards only two types of sugars, glucose and galactose. Too much of a good thing is not good for us.

Reduce the Amount of Circulating Inflammatory Glycoproteins

It is thought that having high levels of circulating inflammatory glycoproteins is what fuels the development of autoimmune disease, heart disease and type 2 diabetes. The C-Reactive Protein test measures this level. Inflammatory glycoproteins also play a role in cancer. If we are sick with a chronic illness or a life-threatening disease we want to get the most healing properties possible from the food we eat. The last thing we want is to give the body fuel that leads to worsening health. Even if we are healthy, eating in an imbalanced way, without enough of some of the essential sugars and healthy glycoproteins, as well as excessive amounts of others, is asking for trouble down the road.

I know it's hard to make these changes. If it's hard for you to give up processed foods and sugar, I'd suggest adding in more of the missing six glyconutrients to your diet. Get your glucose with whole food sources. I'm adding in fresh aloe gel to lemonade that I make with stevia. Ask your naturopath or integrative medicine doctor if that would be good for you. Ask them for other suggestions on the remaining glyconutrients.

The Benefits of Cleansing

There are two important ways that we can improve our health quickly: by doing an intestinal cleanse and changing our diet at least while we are in a healing phase. A cleanse clears out mucus from our intestinal tract. As I mentioned before, mucus is produced to protect our digestive tract from stomach acid which has not been properly neutralized if our bile is of poor quality or is too thick to move from bile duct to gallbladder to small intestine. Cleansing allows us to get the full nutritional benefit of the food we eat. It also sweeps away pockets of bad bacteria that are working against us and attacking the intestinal wall.

The Ayurvedic version allows intestinal repair by eating easy-to-digest food during the cleanse. It simplifies life for the digestive tract so that it can clear away unhealthy cilia and start growing new cilia where damage has occurred.

I'd suggest asking an Ayurvedic, integrative or naturopathic doctor, nutritionist (or oncologist during cancer treatment) if it would be healthy and safe to reduce mucus in the digestive tract as a support for the body. It makes sense also to selectively reduce foods with little nutritional value that are high in histamines. The Ayurvedic cleanses I've done can take as little as three days.

The Lowdown on Histamine

Let's talk about histamine in more depth. As I mentioned earlier, histamine is a neurotransmitter that communicates messages from the body to the brain. It causes an immediate inflammatory response. It's meant to be a red flag to the immune system, notifying the body of any attackers so it can find the location of the problem.

It is meant to send a quick signal and get broken down immediately by DAO (diamine oxidase) which is produced in the intestinal tract. Things can go wrong in the production of DAO if the intestinal tract is not in good health. The following can widen the cell spacing of the gut lining: gluten intolerance, leaky gut, SIBO (small intestinal bacteria overgrowth), intestinal inflammation and/or medication like aspirin, ibuprofen, and some anti-depressants like Cymbalta, Prozac, Zoloft and Effexor. Widened cell spacing allows food particles to escape the digestive tract. Medicines such as some immune modulators, some antiarrhythmics, as well as some antihistamines and histamine blockers can all impair DAO production. As listed earlier, there are lots of foods that contain high levels of histamine. In addition to foods containing high histamine, some foods cause our bodies' mast cells to release histamine as if we were under immune attack. This list includes most citrus fruits, chocolate, cow's milk, papaya, shellfish, strawberries, tomatoes, nuts and wheat germ, along with additives like sulphites, nitrites, glutamate, food dyes and benzoate.

DAO-blocking foods include alcohol, which makes beer and wine a double whammy, since they're high in histamines too. Other DAO blockers are energy drinks, black tea, green tea and matcha.

Stress and Histamine Intolerance

High stress levels could be causing histamine intolerance to dietary histamines. Additionally, our diet may be too high in DAO blockers. I have found that as I have reduced my stress levels and been consistent with yoga and meditation that I have more tolerance for dietary histamines.

Excess Dietary Histamines and the Pain Poor Health Insomnia Cycle

To give you an example about how strongly histamine can affect a person, my wakeup call came after following advice to make homemade yogurt cultured for 24 hours. I had been rebounding in health from all the changes I'd made in my life and by that point I could do hot yoga three times a week. Day One of eating that yogurt, I went into hot yoga and after 15 minutes I had to lie down on my back. I got up after 5 minutes and then had to lie down another 15 minutes. I spent the rest of the class like that. I felt like Superman encountering kryptonite for the first time—I couldn't figure out what had gone wrong! I hadn't learned about histamine at that point. It turns out that the longer we culture a food, the higher the histamine levels. I went back to hot yoga two more times and was weak as a kitten each time. After that last time, I stopped eating yogurt. I went to hot yoga the following day and was as strong as I'd been before eating yogurt; I powered right through the class. And that was the day I decided to boot yogurt from my life until I'm 100% better. If you have leaky gut, it's possible you too might be impacted by histamines without realizing it.

Immune System Overreaction and Histamine Intolerance Response

As I mentioned before, sometimes when I ate salad with a strong vinegar dressing I would start to cough and choke a bit. In the past, I just figured vinegar just hit my windpipe the wrong way, but then I realized it set off a huge immune response that caused so much inflammation that it allowed in the very bacteria or viruses it was trying to defend against. For me, even just one eighth of a teaspoon of vinegary dressing can lead to a sore throat that goes into the common cold and congested sinuses. I bet I am not the only one.

This explains how I could have gotten sick so frequently. We do not have the same reaction to each type of dietary histamine; for me vinegar is the worst offender. If you think histamine could be impacting you, try to figure out which type is the worst for you. That way you can customize your diet to eat as many of the foods you love as you can while minimizing any hardship.

Leaky gut leads to molecules being released into the bloodstream that are intended to stay within the gut. The body makes histamine when this happens. I have a problem with wheat from leaky gut, so when wheat gets into my bloodstream I start to have sinus congestion (histamine leads to mucus being formed in the sinuses). This led me to get chronic sinus infections.

Most people with chronic fatigue syndrome (now called either SEID or M.E./CFS) and Fibromyalgia have the genetic problem of not being able to use some B vitamins unless they are already in a converted, ready-to-use state. The body has to do up to four steps before some B vitamins are ready for use. Fortunately, there are methylated forms of B vitamins available for those who, like me, have an issue.

Unfortunately, rebuilding wellness is complicated and the process can lead to feeling worse initially instead of feeling better right away. It is important to find the right doctor to help. I have found integrative medicine doctors, Ayurvedic doctors, naturopaths and fusion or functional medicine doctors understand this best.

In trying to heal the body once chronic conditions have set in, it is important to repair the gut by following one of the diets such as GAPS or BED or a diet that tries to limit high histamine foods that don't build health. The best way to rebuild our health is through adding bioflavonoids (in other words, not fearing healthy high histamine foods), as Healing Histamine suggests. Unfortunately, these diets don't have much overlap. I suggest that you evaluate your biggest problem; is it intestinal distress or is it pain, fatigue or insomnia? Treat the worst condition first. I'll discuss GAPS and BED later in this chapter.

Oxalates in Food

Oxalate and oxalic acid are organic acids that come from some plants, fungus such as aspergillus and candida, as well as metabolic processes in the body. Oxalates are powerful oxidants that can cause tissue damage, pain and inflammation. Most of us don't have to think twice about oxalates because the flora of the gut will metabolize it or it will pass through the body in the stool. Those of us with inflammation in the gut can absorb damaging levels of oxalates. A healthy person might absorb 1-2% of dietary oxalates and an unhealthy one might absorb 50% of dietary oxalates. *Never cut oxalates out of your diet all at once because it can cause a fatal reaction as the body tries to remove them from where they've been stored.* We need to slowly dial down how much we eat. Here are seven conditions with good reason to avoid oxalates: if you are on the autistic spectrum, if you have digestive issues like leaky gut, if you have fibromyalgia, depression, arthritis, interstitial cystitis (chronic bladder pressure and pain) or vulvodynia (chronic pain in the vulvar region which includes burning or irritation.)

Proper levels of nutrients like calcium are important to help eliminate oxalates safely. This is an area where not a lot of medical research has been done and where there isn't a standard best practices pathway. It's best to get help from an integrative medicine doctor to reduce oxalates. *Proceed with extreme caution!* Dr. Susan Owen is an oxalate researcher recommended by Yasmina Yekelenstam of Healing Histamine. Dr. Owen recommends an online Yahoo! support group called Trying_Low_Oxalates; again, I can't stress enough to please work through something like this with your nutritionist or doctor. The highest levels of oxalates in any food by far are found in spinach, which I have cut out of my diet until I'm completely healed. I've also cut out foods that are considered high in oxalates-- because I don't tend to eat a lot of spinach. I felt that was safe. I have such a restricted diet that I would rather not cut out medium level oxalate foods, but I may try it in the future. I have noticed a significant difference in pain levels with just cutting out high oxalate foods.

Lectins

As I mentioned in Chapter 21, lectins are found in all forms of life. When trying to rebuild our health, it's important to look to avoiding nuts, beans and grains that are not soaked or fermented, or cooked at a specific temperature for a certain length of time. Sally Fallon has a cookbook called *Nourishing Traditions* that is a resource. So is Sandor Katz's book *Wild Fermentation.* There are dozens of cookbooks and blogs out there to help you, but a word of caution: go slow. If you have a leaky gut, these fermented bacteria are getting into your bloodstream and taxing your immune system. Soaking seems like a safer way to go, at least until you've overcome your leaky gut. Research how to prepare foods that are high in lectins—for example, as few as four or five raw kidney beans can trigger lectin poisoning. Red kidney beans can only be safely eaten after having been boiled for 30 minutes and should never be prepared in a slow cooker for that reason, as the temperature never gets high enough. Have a tablespoon of a fermented bean dish, not half a plate. Evaluate how you feel after that tablespoon. If you're experiencing any symptoms of histamine intolerance like headaches, migraines, anxiety, arrhythmia or accelerated heart rate, difficulty falling asleep, dizziness, nausea, vomiting, or hypertension, back off the soaked and fermented food and have a talk with your integrative, naturopathic, or Ayurvedic doctor. Report how you're feeling and ask further advice about how to rebuild gut health.

Glutamic Acid

Glutamic acid is an amino acid found in plant and animal protein. Glutamate is the most common form of glutamic acid in our bodies. Glutamate is a neurotransmitter that is vital to help our brain learn, grow, develop and recall. The issue with glutamate is when it is free –no longer bound in a whole food source—and therefore able to be absorbed rapidly. Free glutamate is found in high concentrations in some natural foods and it is also found in a lot of processed foods. Certain people are more susceptible; namely if you have problems with leaky gut, there is a possibility that low level chronic inflammation could have led to problems with a leaky blood-brain barrier. Additionally, there's a suggestion of genetic susceptibility for kids with autistic spectrum or ADHD, Huntington's Disease and people who suffer from migraines.

Natural sources for free glutamate are matured, cured or preserved foods, such as cheeses like Parmesan and blue cheese and cured meats like salami. Other sources include mushrooms, tomatoes, broccoli, peas, walnuts, grape juice, bone broth as well as long-braised meats, wheat gluten, dairy casein, malted barley, and aged sauces like fish sauce and soy sauce.

Free glutamate in processed foods can be listed in many ways: monosodium or monopotassium glutamate, yeast extract, anything hydrolyzed, autolyzed yeast, textured protein, gelatin, soy protein (both isolate and concentrate), whey protein (both isolate and concentrate), milk powder, carrageenan, kombu and other seaweeds, bouillon, broth, stock, maltodextrin, pectin, citric acid, corn starch, corn syrup, modified food starch, and often flavors, such as "natural vanilla flavor".

Free glutamate is overstimulating to the brain. Some areas of the brain, like the hypothalamus, do not have an impermeable blood brain barrier, according to the American Nutrition Association.

Excess free glutamate can injure and even kill neurons. The ANA says that at least 25% of the US population react to free glutamate from food sources, and these reactions range between mild and transitory to debilitating and life-threatening. A disparate number of disease conditions such as ALS (Lou Gehrig's Disease), Alzheimer's disease, seizures and stroke are associated with glutamate cascade. So are symptoms like tachycardia, hives, diarrhea, chest pain, dizziness, weakness, chills, unusual perspiration, a flushing sensation in the face or chest, tinging, skin rash, stiffness, joint pain, flu-like achiness, extreme rise or drop in blood pressure, sciatica, slurred speech, lethargy, sleepiness, insomnia, runny nose, asthma, shortness of breath, nocturia, (excessive urination at night), mouth lesions, anxiety, panic attacks and depression. Babies and small children are the most vulnerable. While many manufactures removed monosodium glutamate from their food, they often left free glutamic acid such as "autolyzed yeast" and "hydrolyzed vegetable protein" in their products. Symptoms may be immediate or take up to 48 hours to appear.

I must admit I love some processed foods, both for convenience and even taste. In today's busy world, it's hard to be a purist and I don't aim to be. I'm just more careful because of leaky gut issues as I rebuild my health. I also limit them because of my genetic predisposition towards Type 2 diabetes. I'm mindful to enjoy the heck out of them whenever I do indulge.

Candida

I think it's possible that people who are in sympathetic nervous system dominance are more susceptible to candida. Taking a cell wall suppressor (something which prevents candida from forming a cell wall, which makes it more vulnerable to our immune system) is one way to reduce yeast overload. At the same time, it is important to reduce emotional holding patterns and stress levels, as well as to reset the amygdala.

Women going through peri-menopause and menopause are

often under high levels of stress which can cause histamine intolerance. That can sometimes be relieved by reducing our intake of dietary histamines and including more self-care and holistic therapies in our lives. Making sure to take a probiotic while on antibiotics is important to help keep candida in balance, as can keeping sugar intake low and removing other candida-supporting foods from the diet.

BED or GAPS Diet to Starve the Bad Bacteria and Reseed with Good

BED stands for the Body Ecology Diet by Donna Gates. The GAPS Diet is described by Dr. Natasha Campbell-McBride in her *book Gut and Psychology Syndrome.* These diets look to reduce the intake of short chain carbohydrates found in foods which are poorly absorbed in the small intestine. Omnash University in Melbourne, Australia created the term FODMAP to describe these short chain carbohydrates: fermentable oligo-, di-, mono-saccharides and polyols.

FODMAPs are short-chain polymers of fructose called fructans, galactose (galactans), disaccharides (lactose), monosaccharides (fructose) and polyols which are sugar alcohols like sorbitol, mannitol, xylitol and maltitol. FODMAPs can feed any bad bacteria you have in your digestive tract, so it is worth figuring out what kind of FODMAP your bad bacteria like.

It is rare that we have the same reaction to each type of FODMAP because we tend to predominate in a few types of bad bacteria. Each type of short chain carbohydrate is tested in an elimination diet, so we can see which bacteria are causing us digestive distress.

Once we figure it out, we can help reduce the worst offenders by avoiding that type of FODMAP for a certain amount of time. Taking probiotics will help reseed the space left in the digestive tract that the offender occupied. It doesn't have to be perfect; being in better balance will help our bodies heal.

Ultimately, adding nutritionally dense, healthy foods high in bioflavonoids is the way to go daily.

Action steps:

Easy: If you have leaky gut, avoiding multiple high histamine foods at once could reduce how hard your immune system has to work. For example, make it a treat rather than the norm to eat a salad with avocado, aged cheese and balsamic dressing while having a beer. Reduce how often you pair drinking wine while eating a corned beef sandwich, melted cheese and a pickle.

Consider your reaction to high free glutamate foods and take steps to cut back if needed. Read more about the issue at americannutritionassociation.org.

Ask your doctor if it's okay to take a daily probiotic.

Be careful if you have leaky gut, because probiotics are particularly alarming to the body when they circulate in your blood stream. Certain types are better than others, but ultimately let your body be your guide.

Healinghistamine.com has e-cookbooks to give people with histamine issues an idea about how to cook to heal.

Mark Sissman is also concerned with rebuilding gut health and his blog has archives on how to navigate histamine issues. Whether you're on a paleo diet or not, it's a good educational tool. It's at marksdailyapple.com.

Dr. Josh Axe has a good website with lots of educational material focused on using food as medicine. It's full of recipes for rebuilding health. His website is at draxe.com.

Moderate: Try making dietary changes. Buy a cookbook on the subject and see if you can add in some healthy, nutrient-dense foods.

I've been helped by colonic irrigation with a licensed practitioner, at times using hydrogen peroxide, other times chlorophyll, to assist the intestinal tract in healing. The hydrogen peroxide helped reduce bacterial attack and speed up repair. The chlorophyll gave me energy. Ask your doctor if colonic irrigation is safe for you to try.

Harder: Work with an integrative medicine doctor, fusion doctor or naturopath. Dr. Roach is at themidwaycenter.com. Dr. James Pilc's fusion and meditation practice is at completewellnesswny.com. (By the way, he's got a great voice and I enjoy his meditation CD's.) My local doctor, Dr. Lizzie Clapham, is a naturopath and I've gotten a lot of great help from her. She is at pathways2nh.com.

Dr. Sara Whitney has been a huge help for me with cutting edge Lyme treatment. She consults with doctors at the top of their field in Lyme disease and brings both their expertise and hers to Los Angeles. She is at theroxburyinstitute.com.

Find an Ayurvedic doctor and try a cleanse if recommended for you. You can reach Dr. Douillard at lifespa.com.

Chapter 24
Cognitive Hypnotherapy and HeartSpeak

Improve Digestion, Nutritional Absorption, and Internal Repair with Hypnotherapy

I'm writing about cognitive hypnotherapy in this section rather than in the psychology section because of its importance in improving our digestive health. Reworking how we live in the world and our unconscious beliefs is something that a good cognitive hypnotherapist can help us with. While we do so, we are also healing our immune reactions to foods we ate during times of emotional upsets in our lives.

We each come into the world with our unique traits, and pairing a sensitive child with a harsh environment (or even a not particularly sensitive child with a harsh environment) can mean that our fight-or-flight alarms are triggered for the rest of our lives. Even for adults, life events like breaking a bone, the death of a loved one, divorce or job loss can trigger PTSD. We can become sensitized to foods that we eat because our immune system associates the trauma of an event with food that was eaten around the same time. The good news is that it doesn't have to stay this way. Examining our unconscious beliefs, how we interact with our emotions, our self-talk—all of these can be worked with. It's never too late to redo the way we interact with the world. Additionally, despite all the other work I've done, cognitive hypnotherapy helped me quickly release additional deeply-held beliefs that were keeping me from moving forward.

There are a variety of cognitive hypnotherapy programs available online. The one I took was offered by Yasmina Yekelenstam of Healing Histamine, who partnered with a cognitive hypnotherapist, Hazel Gale, to develop a program which decouples those lifelong connections. It's not a cure, but it can help reduce symptoms.

Choose what's right for your Budget and Ability

The Healing Histamine hypnotherapy program was a four-week program with a daily calming meditation to put us in a parasympathetic state. It also had us journaling daily. We were led through the process of examining the first time we felt a particular emotion and what beliefs we'd accepted about ourselves and the world, so that we could change the programming and enlist our internal abilities to heal.

The downside of online cognitive hypnotherapy programs is that they are not tailored to individual needs. For example, looking at the group's Facebook user posts, I could see that some people were unable to start working on the program because their unconscious fears were so triggered. Hazel and Yasmina did a great job of helping people through the process. I confess I was somewhere in the middle on this one—I got several weeks into it and life "suddenly got too busy" to proceed with it. I'm always suspicious that my unconscious fears are stalling my progress when life events step in like that. If you try a group hypnotherapy program and get stalled, you might want to try individual therapy. That said, I was enormously helped by those first two weeks. One of the first things we did was create an "anchor", which is a word or phrase to calm the nervous system down. I still use that anchor when I'm stressed. I did need to get one-on-one help to finish the program.

Another way to Understand Allergies and Asthma Triggers

It's not widely known that our bodies can make connections between food and trauma. The body can develop an autoimmune response to the food we ate at the time when we were traumatized. A lot of people don't realize that this is what allergy is—that there is connection between our emotions and our immune system. The same process causes triggers for asthma too, according to Dr. Buteyko, whom I mentioned in Chapter 15. So, one reason a person might have an inflammatory response to a food could be because when they first ate it, a parent yelled at them harshly, or right after they ate it, they got word that someone in the family had died, or they ate that food and then got bullied in school. It's all completely unconscious.

Going through hypnotherapy can help reset the mind and body to improve our relationship with food, our ability to digest and absorb the nutrients in our food, and our ability to be in a parasympathetic state so we can repair our bodies. Perhaps the result of this might eventually be a reduction in medication, too, but this needs to be worked through with your doctor. Please don't stop taking medications without getting a doctor's approval. Allergies and asthma are life-threatening conditions.

HeartSpeak

Another way into emotions that are stuck is a relatively new program called HeartSpeak. Developed by Dr. Anne Jensen, a clinical researcher with a PhD in Evidence-based Health Care from Oxford University in the UK, she's also been working to show the efficacy of muscle-testing.

HeartSpeak reconnects a client to their emotional mind. It uses muscle testing to determine what needs to be cleared. The client gets detailed information about how to maximize clearing and is led through steps to release the held emotion. I'm mentioning HeartSpeak in this section because I am trying it as part of trying to expand the list of foods I can eat.

To be completely clear, I am not suggesting anyone ever try this with foods they have an anaphylactic reaction to, which are called IgE allergies. I'm only referring to IgG foods, and only under these strict caveats: I've been tested for foods I have an IgG reaction to. Once I've eliminated the foods for long enough that I test as no longer having an IgG sensitivity to eating them, I'm allowed to rotate those foods through my diet. I use HeartSpeak when I'm about to eat a food that I've had an IgG reaction to in the past. I'm doing this in the hope that it helps reduce my body's reaction to the food over time. I'm not suggesting anyone else try this; I'm only telling you what I'm trying. If I find it helpful, I will update this book with that info.

Action Steps:
Easy: try Les Fehmi's Open Focus meditation if you have anxiety, PTSD or histamine issues.

Moderate: get one-on-one help from a cognitive hypnotherapist about whatever issues you are facing. Hazel Gale can be reached at hazelgale.com.

Find a HeartSpeak practitioner and schedule a session. I use HeartSpeak with my coaching clients. Dr. Anne can be reached at heartspeak.com. There are over 300 practitioners in multiple countries as this book goes to press.

Harder: combine cognitive therapy and meditation with dietary changes that your doctor or nutritionist okays.

Take Level 1 and 2 of HeartSpeak to get tools to help your family and friends or to become a practitioner.

Chapter 25
The Power of Intention

A Word about Empaths

People who are traumatized as children have learned to tune in and listen to other people's emotional states before their own, as a way to stay safe. This is called being empathic. The problem is that empaths do not learn to listen to their own internal states, so they are often not sure what they think or believe or feel.

They often find their feelings inconvenient or downright dangerous at times—feelings did not help their survival as children, so they stuffed them. Most likely they don't seem helpful in adulthood either. Anger over their treatment in childhood or as an adult may have endangered them or their relationships and required them to suppress it. Empaths think they can push their feelings aside or bury them because that is what they've always done, and it has always worked.

They tend to repeat the patterns of their childhood and find relationships that echo the problems they encountered as children. Those problems are familiar--and familiar feels safe to the unconscious, even when it isn't safe to the rational mind. Being empathic can be a perfect breeding ground to become codependent.

Empaths can be extroverts or introverts. Introverted empaths can lose their way and remain frozen or trapped by others' needs or fears. The juggling act involved in trying to read mirror neurons in a room full of people is exhausting for them.

On the path back to health, introverted empaths must be aware of their internal state, figure out what emotion they are feeling, and assign that feeling as much value as another person's feelings. In this way, they can break free of co-dependency.

The Aladdin Factor

As Jack Canfield and Mark Victor Hansen say in *The Aladdin Factor*, "The truth is all facts are facts and all events are meaningless. You are the one who makes up the meaning and once you make the event mean something, that meaning becomes an unexamined box that can limit or disempower you." Introverts have a mountain of unexamined boxes which limit and disempower us. It all starts with a willingness to examine a box. You can choose to welcome the opportunity to start examining those boxes. If you do, you'll live life like Bill Murray in the movie *Groundhog Day* after he finally starts giving his life a positive meaning. Everything that has happened to us this far is what was necessary to have us wake up and start taking positive steps. No more beating ourselves up for the-might-have-beens.

Happily Self-Parenting for Life

Start parenting your inner self in a kind way. What we've said to ourselves over the course of a lifetime has likely been far harsher than optimal. As Jack Canfield mentions in *The Success Principles*, according to researchers, we think an average of 50,000 thoughts a day, 80% of which are negative and most of those are about ourselves.

There surely is someone out there whose parents didn't love them, whose friends have never been there for them and have only used them. But telling yourself these types of things is only going to shut you down and paralyze you more because it scares the unconscious. If you have tried the logical and rational left-brained way, telling yourself such dire things and have gotten sick, it makes sense to try a different way. If you live in fear, paralysis, avoidance or anger, try being kind to yourself. You need to positively parent your inner child. Would anyone say tens of thousands of negative things to a three-year-old child every day? If they did, that child would be a wreck.

You are Loved

Try telling yourself for a week that everyone loved you and wanted the best for you to the best of their abilities. Repeat this sentence multiple times a day. If you notice you feel better at the end of the week, continue it. It is ultimately a gift to yourself. You deserve to have it be true. You are worthy. Telling yourself that it is true will free you up to enjoy your life in ways you didn't think possible. Don't you deserve to enjoy your life to the fullest?

Telling yourself what you logically perceive as true is keeping you a victim of your actual parenting. Begin the re-parenting process if you feel in need. If this rings a bell for you, you will need to promise that inner three-year-old that you will take care of him or her, now that you have learned how. Apologize for letting that three-year-old down and tell him or her that you will listen.

Imagine hugging your three-year-old self. Remember how adorable and loving you were. See how worthy you were of love and kindness. You may not have gotten it then but from here on out you can provide it. You can happily and successfully learn to be a better self-parent.

Weekly Self Care

What do you do to help encourage yourself every week? Try taking a bath with Epsom salts (or if pressed for time, a shower with a sugar scrub). Think about all the parts of your body which have helped you, and thank them one by one: from organs to glands, from skin to muscle, from fascia to bones, etc.

Judgments Poison

Become aware of the times that you judge. As Jesus said, "Judge not lest you be judged." While we are wired to be human judgment machines, we don't have to be that way. When we judge others, we wind up being a harsher judge of ourselves than if we try to let go of our judgment of others.

We often internalize the most judgmental adults in our lives as our inner critic when we were young. They live on in how we put ourselves down, and in turn how we focus on others' faults, so that we have relief from judging ourselves. Far better to ease up on the inner critic's hold on you. When that self-judgment shows up, thank it for helping and tell it that you're running the show now.

Experiment with this for yourself and see if it holds true for you. You deserve to be happier. If you believe in God or a universal energy be sure to add that element to your self-talk, reminding yourself that God or The Universe loves you. Even if you do not believe in God or a universal energy, even if your prayer consists of, "Hey _____, I don't believe in you but here's what's going on," (fill in the blank and add a sentence on to it that you are loved by this thing), it can help reduce your stress. If it sounds interesting, you can choose to try it for a week and see if you are happier or calmer. Above all, you still get to be you during this process.

Final Thoughts

As this book winds down, I want to make sure it leaves you with a path out of whatever health issues and/or pain you currently have. You always have the choice to not take any suggestions from this book. It's your decision to make. If you think you'd like to start taking a step, maybe pick an easy one. One easy start down the path back to health is to begin taking a supplement of trace minerals. Another choice might be to start timing when you drink water before meals to aid your stomach acid production.

The important thing is not to load up on too many steps at once. Why not treat yourself kindly? Whether you add the second step in after a week or two, or after a month or two, or six or eight, it is forward momentum and you'll get there.

Give yourself a pat on the back, you have earned it. If you're shy, go on, find somewhere private and give yourself a real pat on the back. Get used to doing silly things like that. You would be amazed at how much it means to your inner child, and really, no one else needs to know. Learn how to muscle test so you can ask your inner child what it wants for breakfast, or to wear for the day, or what way to get exercise.

When somebody first learns how to juggle, they are not using multiple balls at once and expecting to be successful right away. They start simply and get the feel for the first step; then once that is mastered they add another ball. The ones who succeed at juggling are the ones who make the learning process enjoyable by being kind to themselves. Wherever we've succeeded in our lives, it's because either we or someone else in our lives provided a safe space for us to practice mastery until we acquired it. Now that you consciously know that, you can master anything if you are willing to take the time to learn how to provide a safe space for yourself as you practice.

Those who truly succeed in life are the ones who make the learning and living process enjoyable by being kind to themselves. We all need to show ourselves the same courtesy. Once we have set our intention, we should realize its power to carry us through the change. Visualize it often in detail. Reaffirm it regularly and enjoy your best health ever.

Action Steps:
Easy: Read *The Aladdin Factor*, by Jack Canfield and Mark Victor Hansen.

Ask your doctor if it's okay to take trace minerals like what you'd find in health food stores, or Ancient Earth Minerals from bodyecology.com.

Drink eight glasses of water every day, making sure to time it so that you're drinking a glass 15-30 minutes before eating.

Look back through the other chapters at the easy steps and see which appear truly easy to you. Make a list of easy steps for you to take and put them in order of priority so you can add them in whenever it feels right.

Moderate: Make a commitment to stop judging others so harshly. If you are Christian, realize that 'thou shall love thy neighbor as thyself' doesn't mean love the easy people. It means all of them. Every single human being. It's really a way of loving *ourselves*, because the parts of ourselves which we find unlovable are hidden away until other people who are like those 'unlovable' parts trigger us. Often our unconscious reasoning is why should other people get to be like those parts of ourselves that our parents or others shamed us about or punished us for, and so we lash out against other people rather than ourselves or our parents. Instead, by treating others with kindness, we begin to heal our inner child and start rebuilding our health.

Harder: Keep a journal about the emotions you experience. Notice the conclusions you make and how often you are right in predicting how something is going to turn out when you're in the middle of strong emotion. If you're like most people, you're rarely right. Notice if that makes it any easier to let go of your emotions. Remind yourself that research shows mentally bracing for disaster is not effective in actual emergencies. Instead visualize positive outcomes. Allow yourself to be hopeful as you wait for life to play out.

Try getting support for your growth from psychologists and specialized kinesiologists near you.

Learn how to Focus. More info at focusing.org.

Once you've integrated all the lessons you've chosen from this book, I suggest you take stock of your life three or four times a year by looking at the Monday through Friday lessons. On Monday, make sure you've still got flow in your life and that you've taken steps to reduce stress. On Tuesday, ask yourself about your pain levels, etc. Remember that if you've fallen short, that's a judgment, so be sure to give yourself a positive word of encouragement for your intention.

Here is to the miracle you already are, may you come to fully see it for yourself.

Love,
Elizabeth

Appendix
ACE Test *
Finding Your ACE Score
More info available at cdc.gov/ace and acestudy.org.

While you were growing up, during your first 18 years of life:

1.Did a parent or other adult in the household often or very often...
Swear at you, insult you, put you down, or humiliate you? or act in a
way that made you afraid that you might be physically hurt? Yes No
If yes enter 1 _____

2. Did a parent or other adult in the household often or very often...
Push, grab, slap, or throw something at you? or Ever hit you so hard
that you had marks or were injured? Yes No
If yes enter 1 _____

3. Did an adult or person at least 5 years older than you ever... Touch
or fondle you or have you touch their body in a sexual way? or
Attempt or actually have oral, anal, or vaginal intercourse with you?
Yes No
If yes enter 1 _____

4. Did you often or very often feel that ... No one in your family
loved you or thought you were important or special? or Your family
didn't look out for each other, feel close to each other, or support each
other? Yes No
If yes enter 1 _____

5. Did you often or very often feel that ... You didn't have enough to
eat, had to wear dirty clothes, and had no one to protect you? or Your
parents were too drunk or high to take care of you or take you to the
doctor if you needed it? Yes No
If yes enter 1 _____

6. Were your parents ever separated or divorced? Yes No
If yes enter 1 _____

7. Was your mother or stepmother: Often or very often pushed,
grabbed, slapped, or had something thrown at her? or Sometimes,

often, or very often kicked, bitten, hit with a fist, or hit with something hard? or Ever repeatedly hit at least a few minutes or threatened with a gun or knife?   Yes   No

If yes enter 1 _____

8. Did you live with anyone who was a problem drinker or alcoholic or who used street drugs?   Yes No   If yes enter 1 _____

9. Was a household member depressed or mentally ill, or did a household member attempt suicide? Yes   No   If yes enter 1 _____

10. Did a household member go to prison?   Yes   No

If yes enter 1 _____

Now add up your "Yes" answers: _____ This is your ACE Score.

*Remember that we are not victims of our childhood. Awareness of the issue leads us to develop a toolbox to reset our nervous systems, which leads to post-traumatic growth and resilience. You can do it!

Bibliography / Recommended Reading

Adams, Case PhD   *Natural Solutions for Food Allergies and Intolerance*

Agus, David MD *The End of Illness*

Amand, R. Paul MD   *What Your Doctor May Not Tell You About Fibromyalgia*

Amen, Daniel MD   *Healing ADD*

Amen, Daniel MD   *Change Your Brain, Change Your Body*

Amen, Daniel MD   *Use Your Brain to Change Your Life*

Arrowsmith Young, Barbara   *The Woman Who Changed Her Brain*

Ball, Ron   *Freedom at Your Fingertips*

Barnes, John   *Healing Ancient Wounds*

Bennett-Goleman, Tara   *Mind Whispering*

Berceli, David Phd   *The Revolutionary Trauma Release Process*

Blaich, Dr. Robert   *Your Inner Pharmacy*

Bolte Taylor, Dr. Jill   *My Stroke of Insight*

Boyle, Dr. Neil   *Why Be In Pain?*

Brostoff, Jonathan MD   *Food Allergies and Food Intolerance*

Brown, Brene   *Daring Greatly*

Brown, Brene   *The Gifts of Imperfection*

Brown, Brene   *Rising Strong*

Browning, Tovi   *Gentle Miracles: Holistic Pulsing*

Brownstein, David MD   *Salt Your Way to Health*

Cain, Susan   *Quiet*

Cameron, Julia   *The Artist's Way*

Campbell-McBride, Dr. Natasha   *Gut and Psychology Syndrome*

Canfield, Jack   *The Aladdin Factor*

Canfield, Jack   *Chicken Soup for the Soul Series*

Canfield, Jack   *Tapping into Ultimate Success*

Capacchione, Lucia PhD   *Recovery of Your Inner Child*

Carlin, Dr. Debra   *Build the Strength Within*

Carlson, Neil   *Foundations of Physiological Psychology*

Carrigan, Catherine   *Unlimited Energy Now*

Chaitow, Leon   *Fibromyalgia Syndrome*

Challem, Jack *The Inflammation Syndrome*
Chilton, Floyd PhD *Inflammation Nation*
Chilton, Floyd PhD *Win the War Within*
Cohen, Dr. Michael *Feel it? Heal it*
Cole, Jonathan *Pride and a Daily Marathon*
Cooley, Bob *Resistance Flexibility 1.0*
Covell, Cathy *Feeling Your Way Through*
Cryder, Chad *Men are DAWGS and Women are CATS: A Field Guide for Human Relationships*
Csikzentmihalyi, Mihaly PhD *Finding Flow*
D'Adamo, Dr. Peter *Eat Right 4 Your Type*
Dahlin, Dondi *The Five Elements: Understand Yourself and Enhance Your Relationships with the Wisdom of the World's Oldest Personality Type System*
Davis, Adelle *Let's Get Well*
Davis, Adelle *Let's Eat Right to Keep Fit*
Dennison, Paul & Gail *Brain Gym ® Teachers Edition*
DeSalvo, Louise *Writing as a Way of Healing*
Doidge, Norman MD *The Brain That Changes Itself*
Douillard, Dr. John *Body, Mind, Sport*
Douillard, Dr. John *Eat Wheat*
Douillard, Dr. John *The 3 Season Diet*
Douillard, Dr. John *Colorado Cleanse*
Eden, Donna *The Little Book of Energy Medicine*
Fehmi, Les PhD *Dissolving Pain*
Feldenkrais, Moshe *Awareness Through Movement*
Feldenkrais, Moshe *Master Moves*
Fields, Jonathan *Uncertainty*
Forbes, Bo *Yoga for Emotional Balance*
Ford, Debbie *The Dark Side of the Light Chasers*
Fredrickson, Barbara PhD *Positivity*
Gendlin, Eugene *Focusing*
Gilbert, Daniel *Stumbling on Happiness*
Gilbert, Elizabeth *Big Magic*

Gilbert, Elizabeth *Eat Pray Love*

Goleman, Daniel *Social Intelligence*

Gottchall, Elaine *Breaking the Vicious Cycle*

Hannaford, Carla *Smart Moves: Why Learning Isn't All in Your Head*

Hartwig, Dallas & Melissa *It Starts with Food*

Haynes, Anthony *Food Intolerance Bible*

Heath, Chip & Dan *Switch*

Heller, Laurence PhD *Healing Developmental Trauma*

Hitzmann, Sue *The MELT Method*

Hubert, Bill *Bal-A-Vis-X*

Hyman, Mark MD *The Ultramind Solution*

Ingebretson, Susan *Fibrowhyalgia*

Ingram, Dr. Cass *The Respiratory Solution*

Ivker, Robert *Sinus Survival*

Jackson Nakazawa, Donna *Childhood Interrupted*

Jackson Nakazawa, Donna *The Last Best Cure*

Kalsched, Donald PhD *The Inner World of Trauma*

Kaplan, Melvin *Seeing Through New Eyes*

Kaplan, Melvin *The Secrets in Their Eyes*

Karnis, Joyce *Comprehensive Myofascial Self Treatment*

Kerson, Dr. Don *Getting Unstuck: Unraveling the Knot of Depression, Attention and Trauma*

Keyes, Ken *The Power of Unconditional Love*

Kraftsow, Gary *Yoga for Transformation*

Levine, Peter PhD *Waking the Tiger*

Lipski, Elizabeth PhD *Digestive Wellness*

Lozoff, Bo *We're All Doing Time*

Masgutova, Svetlana *Masgutova Method*

Meyer, Joyce *Living Beyond Your Feelings*

Mullin, Gerard MD *The Inside Tract*

Mullin, Gerard MD Integrative Gastroenterology

Musil, Donna *Brats: Our Journey Home (DVD Documentary*)

Neff, Kristen PhD *Self-Compassion*

Nelson, Dr. Bradley   *The Emotion Code*

Northrup, Christianne MD   *Goddesses Never Age*

Oleska, Paula   *Your Secret Brain- DVD*

Ornstein, Robert   *The Right Mind: Making Sense of the Hemispheres*

Pagano, John   *One Cause Many Ailments: Leaky Gut Syndrome*

Pennebaker, James PhD   *Opening Up: The Healing Power of Confiding in Others*

Perl, Sondra   *Felt Sense: Writing with the Body*

Perlmutter, David   *Brain Maker*

Pert, Candace PhD   *Molecules of Emotion*

Ratey, John MD   *Spark*

Rimland, Bernard   *Dislogic Syndrome*

Roach, Dr. Jim   *God's House Calls: Finding God Through my Patients*

Robbins, John   *Reclaiming Our Health*

Rock, David   *Your Brain at Work*

Rome, David   *Your Body Knows the Answer*

Sarnow, Dr John   *The Divided Mind*

Seligman, Martin PhD   *Authentic Happiness*

Seligman, Martin PhD   *Flourish*

Seligman, Martin PhD   *Positive Psychology*

Shimoff, Marci   *Happy for No Reason*

Shimoff, Marci   *Love for No Reason*

Shumway-Cook, Anne   *Motor Control Theory and Practical Applications*

Simon, Bebe   *How I Teach Focusing: Discovering the Gift of Your Inner Wisdom*

Singer, Michael   *The Untethered Soul: The Journey Beyond Yourself*

Solden, Sari   *Women with Attention Deficit Disorder*

Stone, Hal & Sidra   *Embracing Ourselves*

Stutz, Phil   *The Tools*

Tanner Boll, Pamela   *Who Does She Think She Is? (DVD*

Documentary)

Thie, Dr. John and Matthew   *Touch for Health: The Complete Edition*

Truman, Karol   *Feelings Buried Alive Never Die*

Truman, Karol   *Healing Feelings from Your Heart*

Van Vorous, Heather   *Help for IBS*

Wangyal, Tenzin (Rinpoche)   *Healing With Form, Energy and Light*

Wangyal, Tenzin (Rinpoche)   *Sound Healing (Book and DVD)*

Warner, Priscilla   *Learning to Breathe: My Yearlong Quest to Bring Calm to my Life*

Weill, Andrew MD   *Spontaneous Healing*

Wells, Steve   *Enjoy Emotional Freedom*

Zukav, Gary   *The Seat of the Soul*

Zukav, Gary   *Soul to Soul*